The Fiber Prescription

The Fiber Prescription

Myron Winick, M.D.
with William Proctor

FAWCETT COLUMBINE
New York

A Fawcett Columbine Book
Published by Ballantine Books
Copyright © 1992 by Myron Winick, M.D.
and William Proctor

Grateful acknowledgment is made to the following for permission to reprint previously published material:

The American Dietetic Association: Fiber and Calorie Table for Common Foods is reprinted from the *Journal of the American Dietetic Association,* June 1986.

George A. Bray: Nomogram for determining body mass index reprinted from *The International Journal of Obesity.* Copyright 1978 by George A. Bray. Used by permission.

National Academy Press: Table listing desirable body mass index in relation to age reprinted from *Diet and Health: Implications for Reducing Chronic Disease Risk.* Copyright © 1989 by the National Academy of Sciences. Published by National Academy Press, Washington, D.C.

Plenum Publishing Corp. and Hans N. Englyst: Charts showing soluble and insoluble fiber content and other ingredients in selected foods adapted from "Measurement of Dietary Fiber as Nonstarch Polysaccharides" by Hans N. Englyst and John H. Cummings in *Dietary Fiber: Basic and Clinical Aspects* edited by George V. Vahouny and David Kritchevsky, Plenum Publishing, 1986.

Library of Congress Catalog Card Number: 92-90188
ISBN: 0-449-90450-4

Cover photograph by David Spindell

Manufactured in the United States of America
First Edition: August 1992
10 9 8 7 6 5 4 3 2 1

The authors would like to offer special thanks to Diane C. Darcy, M.S., R.D., who was the nutrition consultant on the recipes.

Contents

The Fiber Prescription

1

What Is the Fiber Prescription?

One of the most ancient staples of the human diet, fiber has gained a new popularity in the last two decades—and rightly so. Far from being a hollow, trendy vogue in nutrition, this food has demonstrated its power to reduce the risks of serious health conditions such as heart disease, colon cancer, diverticulitis, constipation, obesity, and diabetes.

How can you maximize its protective potential?

The first step is to eliminate the confusion surrounding the subject. Nutrition in general, and fiber in particular, can be baffling. Several times a week we read or hear news reports from some expert or medical researcher about how a particular food may be the cure-all for a certain disease. Yet sometimes the very next day another expert contradicts the first one.

How can we cut through this quandary? Fortunately, there is a simple *fiber prescription* that focuses on the basic facts about fiber that are currently known and are unlikely to change. The main goal of this book is to present this fiber prescription as a simple and practical action plan that you can begin to use in your kitchen *tonight*. In fact, the fiber prescription is so simple that you can actually change your *next meal* for the better this way:

Simply eat more whole-grain products, fruits, or vegetables—such as whole meal bread, apples, pears, strawberries, bananas, broccoli, brussels sprouts, carrots, potatoes, dried peas, and baked and kidney beans. Each of these contains plenty of fiber that can help you on more than one health front.

Another simple but absolutely essential rule: Eat high-fiber dishes regularly. Sprinkling a little high-fiber product here and there on your plate just won't do; a more thorough eating plan is required for maximum protection of your health and life. In short, fiber must become the centerpiece of every meal.

Of course, to take full advantage of fiber, it's essential to go into more detail. For example, you must grasp how the two main types of fiber operate as a protective cloak in the body. In brief, the two types are:

• *Insoluble fiber*, which can be found in such foods as wheat bran cereals, whole wheat spaghetti, and raw cabbage. Insoluble fiber gets its name from the fact that it does not dissolve in water, as well as in the liquid environment of the stomach and intestines.

• *Soluble fiber*, which is present in such items as oatmeal, oat bran, and dried beans. Soluble fiber *does* dissolve in water, as well as in the gastrointestinal tract.

As you get a firmer idea about which foods contain fiber—and how that fiber can work to bolster various aspects of your health—you'll be ready to design your own individual strategy for incorporating more high-fiber foods into your basic daily food plan.

Consider, for instance, the experience of these people, who discovered how well a sound, fiber-based nutritional strategy can work.

Item #1: A Weapon Against Heart Disease.

A blood test for lipid levels revealed that John, a 38-year-old businessman, had a total cholesterol reading of 235 milligrams per deciliter (mg/dl). Recent medical recommendations say that for the best protection against atherosclerosis (clogging of the arteries by fatty substances in the blood) someone his age should have cholesterol levels below 200. According to one interpretation of leading scientific studies, every 1 percent above 200 raises the person's risk of heart disease by 2 percent.

John had already adjusted his diet by eliminating eggs, cheese, and ice cream. Through these changes, he had lowered his total cholesterol from a high of 265 to the current measurement of 235. But his doctor quite correctly wanted him to lower the cholesterol even more. The prescription: a significant increase in the proportion of soluble fiber in John's diet, including foods such as oat bran, corn bran, and dried beans. (Remember, soluble fiber dissolves in water and in the gastrointestinal tract.)

So John began to eat oatmeal for breakfast, oat bran and corn bran muffins during meals and for snacks, and more beans such as lentils, which are high in soluble fiber. He did continue to eat many of the other dishes that had been a regular part of his diet, such as various meats and vegetables. But he ended up consuming a smaller proportion of these foods than before. Why? His new approach to nutrition caused him to *substitute* the high-fiber foods for many of his old favorites, including meats and sweets that contained a high percentage of saturated fat.

As a result of this new way of eating, John experienced a dramatic change in his cholesterol. Specifically, his reading dropped to 195 mg/dl, or below that critical 200 mark that so many experts now recommend as the target.

Various studies have shown that with a significant increase in the consumption of certain soluble fibers, such as oat bran, many people can expect a decrease in cholesterol of 5 to 10 percent. The soluble fiber apparently binds a certain amount of the body's cholesterol and carries it out of the body as waste through the intestines. In John's case, that would have meant a drop of about 24 mg/dl, or a new total reading of 211.

But in addition to the independent action of the soluble fiber, John's diet had shifted so that the extra fiber was pushing out some of his other regular foods, including those containing saturated fats. Saturated fat—even if it doesn't contain cholesterol—may still elevate the levels of cholesterol in the blood. So the lesser amounts of saturated fat in John's diet helped to reduce his total cholesterol further to 195 mg/dl.

By focusing on fiber, then, John achieved a significant reduction in his risk for heart disease.

Item #2: A Counter to Cancer.

Andy, a 55-year-old public relations representative, was worried because he had a strong history of colon cancer in his family. His father had died from the disease while in his early fifties, and his older brother had already had a premalignant polyp removed from the large intestine.

So far, various exams, including a sigmoidoscopy, showed that Andy's intestinal tract was "clean." But understandably, he was concerned that within another decade he might find that cancer had appeared in his colon. So he asked his doctor for advice on lowering his risk for this disease.

"The best medicine for you right now is to increase your consumption of insoluble fiber and decrease your total fat intake," the physician advised. These two factors—a diet high in insoluble fiber and low in total fats—have been associated in many studies with a lower incidence of colon cancer. As a matter of fact, colon cancer is the third most common cancer among Americans, but it's rare among Africans and other peoples whose diets are high in insoluble fibers.

The doctor also pointed out that one of the best sources of insoluble fiber is wheat bran. Yet adequate amounts of this food can usually be taken in only by eating a cereal high in insoluble fiber every morning. So Andy shifted from his usual breakfast of bacon or sausage and eggs to a meal consisting of one of the standard wheat bran cereals, with skim milk and a sizable quantity of fruit.

Fortunately, Andy was a motivated, disciplined dieter. Because he knew that he might be at higher risk for colon cancer than the average person, he was willing to make changes in his eating habits in an effort to lower that risk.

Also, Andy believed in undergoing regular annual medical exams. Consequently, his doctor was able to monitor his health closely over a period of years.

During the next twelve years, Andy's exams continued to show no trace of cancer. Now 57 years old, he seems to have a bright outlook for continued good health.

It's possible, of course, that Andy would never have gotten cancer, even with his old high-fat, low-fiber diet. On the other hand, there's little doubt that his risk of cancer was lowered by eating more insoluble fiber and less fat. The main lesson for us: A person like Andy can tip the scales of cancer risk in his favor by shifting to insoluble-fiber foods.

Item #3: An All-Natural Laxative.

Anna, a 52-year-old attorney, had suffered from constipation much of her adult life. She had tried all sorts of over-the-counter laxative remedies to relieve her condition, and for a while several of them worked.

Before long, as her body became more accustomed to the medications, their effectiveness decreased. Also, she became almost totally dependent on the drugs to have a bowel movement.

Finally, a nutritionist friend suggested that the main source of her problem might be her diet. She was eating relatively large quantities of high-protein foods, such as chicken and steaks, but very few foods containing bran. At her friend's suggestion, Anna shifted to a high-fiber diet—with a result that changed her life.

Over a period of just a few weeks, the natural ability of her intestines to move waste materials through and out of her system returned. Within two months, Anna could hardly remember what it had been like to be constipated!

For most people, over-the-counter laxatives simply aren't necessary to remedy constipation. All that's usually required is for the person suffering from this condition to increase the amount of fiber intake.

Constipation is almost totally absent in populations that consume a high-fiber diet. The reason? The content of the intestines becomes softened by the accumulation of water that is trapped by the fiber. With this softening, the pressure within the colon is reduced, and the natural ability of the large intestines to move waste materials along the intestinal canal is enhanced.

Item #4: A Key to Successful Weight Control.

Jenny had been trying for years to lose an excess thirty pounds, but to no avail. No matter what diet she attempted, she failed.

Sometimes, she would manage to lose about ten pounds, and once she almost made fifteen. But then, within a few months, she would be right back up to her old weight.

Finally, however, she stumbled onto a surprisingly little-known secret for weight loss—a variation on what I advocate as my high-fiber diet plan. As a result of this diet, Jenny lost those thirty pounds and even a few more in only twelve weeks. And she *kept* them off!

Specifically, Jenny filled her daily menus with high-fiber foods, much as I've recommended in the food plans in this book. As she ate more high-fiber foods, she found she had less room for the extra calories that accompany fatty and sugary dishes.

Jenny even found that she could go into a fast-food restaurant and come out with many fewer calories than she had consumed during her heavier days. Her approach: She would first order salad dishes, fresh fruit, and other items that are high in fiber and lower in calories. As a result, she always found that she had little room for foods that tended to break her diet.

Similar stories could be told of those who have used fiber to lower their risk for diverticulosis and diverticulitis. Diverticulosis, which involves a weakening of the wall of the large intestine, afflicts more than 20 percent of people over age 65, as well as many younger men and women. In a variation on this condition, food or other material and bacteria can sometimes cause an intestinal infection known as diverticulitis.

The answer to this problem? Again, a high-fiber diet, with an emphasis on cereal brans, will reduce the risk of diverticulosis and the ultimate threat, diverticulitis.

Despite the burgeoning list of such success stories, fiber remains in many ways a mystery. Designing a practical high-fiber eating program continues to be a challenge to scientists as well as family meal planners. Concerned consumers frequently pose questions like these:

• What exactly is fiber?
• By what mechanisms do the different types of fiber achieve their health benefits?
• What are the different types of fiber—and which foods contain them?
• How do you measure the fiber content of ordinary foods? Is there an easy or at least a *workable* way for consumers to do this?

In answering such questions, we'll begin to unveil the mystery of fiber. In the process, you'll gain practical and useful knowledge as you prepare to design your own individual diet.

THE END OF THE CONFUSION ABOUT FIBER

What is fiber?

It's not easy to define fiber in succinct, easy-to-under-

10

stand terms. In fact, the difficulty in defining this food is one of the main reasons it remains such a mystery.

In general, fiber is included with vegetables and other foods classified as carbohydrates, as opposed to those comprised of protein or fat.

But fiber is a special kind of carbohydrate. One common definition—a *physiologic* understanding that focuses on the functioning of the intestines and other bodily organs and tissues during digestion—is that fiber is a natural component of plant food which cannot be broken down by the enzymes in the human digestive tract.

Unfortunately, this relatively simple definition falls short. For one thing, fiber is too complex a food to be described entirely in broad terms by what happens in the digestive tract. Also, it's impossible to measure the fiber content of foods by relying merely on the physiologic definition. Yet the measurement of fiber is essential if the consumer hopes to make intelligent choices in the supermarket.

In an attempt to be more precise, scientists have offered a *chemical* definition of fiber—and this is where the mystery surrounding fiber deepens.

Chemists prefer to describe fiber as the sum of a variety of chemical substances in the plant walls and cells. These include insoluble parts of the plant wall, many of which are known by the general term *cellulose*. Wheat bran falls into this category.

Another chemical component of fiber includes soluble parts and secretions of the plant cells, with such exotic names as gums and mucilages. The fiber in oat and corn bran and in various dried beans would be included here.

Still another chemical classification of fibers is the so-called pectic substances, which may be found in citrus fruits, apples, and sugar beets. Other fibers that include a material called hemicellulose may be either soluble or insoluble in water.

Now, I realize that this is not the place for a chemistry lesson, but it is important for you to understand at the very outset that we're dealing with a very complex topic that presents mysteries even for seasoned scientists.

For example, there's no easy way to subject the many foods you eat to precise chemical testing that can tell you exactly how much of each type of fiber these foods contain. The difficulty in measuring fiber and communicating those measurements in simple terms is reflected in the fact that many food labels in supermarkets don't contain a breakdown of the different types of fiber.

Some consumers, for instance, are mainly interested in the fibers that will help prevent constipation or colon cancer—that means primarily insoluble fibers, such as those with a great deal of cellulose. Other consumers, in their effort to lower the risk of heart disease, will be more concerned with cholesterol-reducing soluble fibers.

In many cases, food labels don't distinguish between the two types of fiber. They'll just have a general "fiber content" entry on the label, and the consumer who lacks an adequate understanding of fiber will be left confused. More often than not, he or she will choose the high-fiber food with the wrong chemical components.

As we move through this book, I'll be shedding more light on this mysterious chemical side of the fiber question. By the time you're finished, you should be in a position to pick the foods with the fiber you need, regardless of what the store labels say—or don't say.

THE FIBER PRESCRIPTION
IN A NUTSHELL

Although this book is devoted to explaining the fiber prescription, I want to introduce you now to several basic principles that will constantly recur as we move from topic to topic, and from fiber to fiber.

Principle #1:

It all begins with learning the fundamental facts about fiber.

The effective use of fiber is rooted in your ability to acquire a deeper understanding of what fiber is, how it works, and what kinds of high-fiber foods are best for you. For example, you should know how to identify products with soluble and insoluble fiber, regardless of the lack of information on food labels, and then be able to work those foods in appropriate proportions into your daily menus. You can't make intelligent selections for your dinner table if you lack a knowledge of the basic facts.

Principle #2:

Fiber must become a basic part of your diet, not a "nutritional Band-Aid."

Too often I've encountered people who think that all they need to do to get significant benefits from fiber is to sprinkle a little granola on their food. In fact, scientific studies have shown that to experience the full effect of fiber, it's necessary to eat this food in larger quantities than sprinkling will allow. And that means making it an integral part of your diet.

For example, one 1989 study published in *The Journal of the National Cancer Institute* focused on the protective qualities of All-Bran for colon cancer. One half of the participants were given two full servings of All-Bran, containing 22.5 grams of fiber a day, or about twice what the average American now eats. The other half consumed a comparable amount of a low-fiber cereal. The results: Those eating the high-fiber cereal experienced a shrinking in size and number of polyps in the rectum, while those eating the low-fiber cereal experienced no such shrinkage.

As for the ability of oat bran to lower cholesterol, another study showed that several muffins a day—containing about 100 grams of fiber—are necessary to achieve a 5 to 10 percent lowering of this lipid in the bloodstream.

Obviously, eating fiber in these quantities requires some serious meal planning and can't be accomplished by a nutritional quick fix.

Principle #3:

Learn to substitute high-fiber foods for those with less nutritional value.

One of the main benefits of foods high in fiber is that they're often quite pleasant-tasting and filling, and thus can be eaten in place of those that are less good for you.

For example, eating a well-rounded high-fiber diet instead of high-fat dishes can accomplish a number of goals:

• First, you'll lower your risk of heart disease through the intake of soluble fibers, which reduces your cholesterol level. (Remember, soluble fibers, which dissolve in water, can be found in abundance in such foods as oat bran, oatmeal, and dried beans and peas.)

• Second, you'll tend to consume fewer calories and thus be more likely to lose weight. For example, 1 gram of fat carries 9 calories, while one gram of a carbohydrate-accompanying fiber contains only 4 calories. (The fiber itself contains no calories.)

• Third, taking in more insoluble fibers and fewer foods high in saturated fat will lower your risk of colon cancer in two ways—through the action of the fiber and the absence of the fat. (Insoluble fiber, which goes through the digestive tract intact, is present in such foods as wheat bran cereals, whole meal products, cabbage, and broccoli.)

Principle #4:

Know when enough is enough.

Like all good things, fiber should be consumed in significant but *reasonable* quantities. In this book, I advocate a well-balanced diet, with fiber occupying a large but not overbearing role in daily menus. Fiber can certainly do a great deal of good for you, but it's also necessary to take in various vitamins, minerals, and other nutrients that may not be found in sufficient quantities in high-fiber foods.

For example, you need at least 800 to 1,000 milligrams of calcium a day to maintain bone strength. Yet it's next to impossible to get this amount of calcium without relying on dairy products like milk (including skim milk), cheese, or yogurt, which are not high in fiber. (If you're lactose intolerant—that is, if you have adverse reactions to the milk sugars in dairy products—you may have to rely in part on calcium supplements such as calcium carbonate or calcium citrate. See your physician for instructions.)

It's even possible to "overdose" on fiber, in the sense that eating too much may have a negative impact on your comfort level and even your health. One of the most common problems for those who go on a high-fiber diet too quickly is an uncomfortable increase in gas or, in some cases, diarrhea. Also, an overabundance of fiber can bind, and eliminate from your system too much of such nutrients as iron, calcium, and zinc.

In brief, I recommend that the average adult consume about 20 to 30 grams of all types of fibers a day, though some vegetarians may take in up to 50 grams daily without ill effects. In contrast, the average American eats about 10 grams a day.

In the following chapters, I'll provide you with all the facts and guidance you need to make fiber a priority in your life. Each chapter will focus on a particular set of health concerns. In most situations, I'll first illustrate the concern—such as high cholesterol, cancer, constipation, or obesity—with a practical example. Then I'll give you all the relevant technical information you need to understand how fiber can act to protect your health. Finally, you'll be provided with some practical tips on designing your daily menus to accommodate the principles discussed in the chapter.

At the end of the book, you'll find a comprehensive set of high-fiber menus and recipes. These will enable you to make the fiber prescription a pivotal, permanent part of your life.

With this basic road map in mind, let's move to the first stop on our exploration of how fiber can work wonders for you and your family. We'll examine how high-fiber foods can be a worthy weapon in the war against excess cholesterol.

2

A Worthy Weapon in the War Against Cholesterol

Maggie was shocked when she learned the status of her cholesterol after a routine blood test for an insurance policy.

The lab report showed that her total cholesterol was 290 milligrams per deciliter (mg/dl), a figure that placed her at very high risk for heart disease. Furthermore, her "good" cholesterol—the subcomponent of cholesterol known as high-density lipoprotein (HDL)—was relatively low at 38 mg/dl. Various studies have shown that high HDLs are associated with protection against heart disease, while low HDLs are linked to a higher risk. For a woman her age, 47 years, Maggie's HDL result should have been at least 50, and preferably 60 or above.

After evaluating her blood tests, the insurance company determined that Maggie would not qualify for a "preferred risk" policy, which would have carried substantially lower premiums than the "standard" policy she was issued. This decision upset her, but she was even more disturbed by the health implications of her cholesterol readings.

Maggie consulted with a cardiologist and learned that her high, unbalanced cholesterol was placing her at high risk for cardiovascular disease, including a possible heart attack or stroke. Specifically, she was advised that her total cholesterol should be lowered to 200 or below, and that a "bad" cholesterol subcomponent in her blood, known as low-density lipoprotein (LDL), should be below 125 mg/dl, if possible, instead of the 220 it currently registered.

Deeply concerned about this threat to her health, Maggie resolved to follow to the letter an initial nondrug strategy that her doctor recommended. "We may be able to take care of this thing with a proper diet and exercise," he said. "Then, if that doesn't work, we'll have to try some cholesterol-lowering drugs."

He explained that the four major risk factors for heart disease are cigarette smoking, hyperlipidemia (high blood fats, mainly cholesterol), hypertension, and diabetes, with obesity and sedentary living being important related risk factors. In Maggie's case, the main problem seemed to be the hyperlipidemia; in addition, she was about ten pounds overweight and was leading a relatively inactive lifestyle.

The nondrug program Maggie was placed on included a low-fat diet, which reduced her total fat intake from 40 percent of total calories to less than 30 percent. Also, she began taking a brisk half-hour walk four days a week.

The diet Maggie went on was quite high in fiber, especially soluble fiber. Some of the foods on her daily menus included fresh fruits, vegetables, legumes, oat bran (in the form of muffins and oatmeal), and barley.

This meal plan attacked her cholesterol problem from different directions:

• First, the increase in high-fiber foods acted as a substitute for high-fat foods. By eating more vegetables, grains, and fruits, Maggie automatically had less room for the bacon, eggs, and fatty meats she had consumed before.

• Second, the soluble fiber in these foods bound the cholesterol in her intestinal tract and, as a result, lowered the total cholesterol in her blood. (More on this momentarily.)

• Finally, the carbohydrate-based fruits, vegetables, and breads that contained the soluble fiber carried fewer calories than the fats Maggie had been eating. (Each gram of fat contains about 9 calories, while each gram of carbohydrate contains only 4 calories.) Consequently, Maggie took in fewer calories and in just a few weeks dropped those ten extra pounds.

What did this program do for Maggie's cholesterol problem? The final result was dramatic. Her total cholesterol plummeted to about 200 mg/dl within three months. Furthermore, the LDL ("bad") cholesterol level moved below the 125 threshold that the doctor had wanted.

In addition, the increased physical activity in the walking program brought the HDL ("good") cholesterol level up to 52. (Note: The HDL level typically isn't responsive to any dietary manipulation, but in many people this subcomponent will move up with an increase in endurance exercise.)

Not everyone will have the overwhelmingly positive response to dietary and lifestyle adjustment that Maggie enjoyed. But many will, and for those people a natural, high-soluble-fiber approach can eliminate any need for cholesterol-lowering drugs, with their various side effects.

THE BASELINE PRINCIPLE

Despite the volumes that have been written on the subject, cholesterol is still one of the most misunderstood medical topics among lay people.

Many, for example, believe that your cholesterol level depends almost entirely on what you eat. In fact, though, the level usually depends on how much your liver (and to a much smaller degree, other parts of the body) produces. Most of the cholesterol in the average person is manufactured inside the body, so there are definite limits on the impact of any dietary restrictions.

Exactly how much cholesterol does your body produce? Or to put this another way, what percentage of the cholesterol in your blood is the result of what your liver is manufacturing?

A common estimate is that 70 to 80 percent of your total blood cholesterol comes from inside the body and about 20 to 30 percent from outside, dietary sources. Again, such generalizations can be misleading.

You see, a person with a genetic problem of cholesterol management may have a far greater proportion of cholesterol floating around in the blood than a person with normal genetic mechanisms. Similarly, a person on a high-fat diet may have relatively more blood cholesterol than a person on a low-fat diet.

I prefer to think in terms of a baseline cholesterol range for body-produced cholesterol. Specifically, if all cholesterol and saturated fats were eliminated from the diet, the average person would still have a cholesterol reading in the range of 120 to 150 mg/dl. This means that the body is going to produce that level of cholesterol in the blood *regardless* of diet. Studies on vegetarians who have almost eliminated cholesterol and fats from their diet reveal that they have cholesterol levels in this very range.

This baseline principle means that if your cholesterol reading is 200—and you're a person with normal blood-fat mechanisms—about 150 mg/dl of that cholesterol is coming from inside the body, and about 50 mg/dl is coming from the diet. If your cholesterol reading is 250, 100 mg/dl comes from diet and 150 mg/dl comes from the body (mainly the liver).

One of the most common exceptions to the baseline principle of body-produced cholesterol involves a recently researched phenomenon called receptors, or hooklike devices on cells that "pull" cholesterol out of the bloodstream into the cells. The cells need cholesterol to perform important building functions; that's the main reason why the liver produces cholesterol, regardless of whether or not we bring it into the body through our food.

In some people, however, the receptors on the cells don't work properly. Or they don't work at all. So certain types of cholesterol floating around in the bloodstream fail to be "hooked" into the cells. Consequently, some cholesterol continues to move freely about and eventually becomes lodged in the walls of blood vessels.

As more and more of these cholesterol molecules (and their accompanying protein "garbage") become lodged in vessel walls, they build up to form an obstruction called plaque. The growing plaque progressively narrows the vessels as part of the process known as atherosclerosis, or "hardening of the arteries." This clogging of the arteries, which is most dangerous in the vessels leading to the heart, is the most common cause of heart disease and heart attacks.

But improperly functioning receptors aren't the only source of excess cholesterol. Another danger is that too much cholesterol may come in by way of the diet. The result may be high levels of serum (blood) cholesterol, over and above the baseline cholesterol produced by the body.

How can diet affect cholesterol level?

Cutting back on high-cholesterol foods, such as eggs, whole milk, and cheeses, can reduce cholesterol levels significantly. At the same time, an extremely important factor in cholesterol is the amount of fat, especially saturated fat, that a person consumes.

In general, there are three types of fat in your food: monounsaturated, polyunsaturated, and saturated. They get their names from their differing chemical structures.

Monounsaturated fats (which may be either solid or liquid at room temperature) are thought to be better for your health than saturated fats because they have been associated with lower levels of heart disease. Polyunsaturated fats (which are usually liquid at room temperature) are also preferred over the saturated type.

Saturated fats (which are usually solid at room temperature) have been associated with higher levels of blood cholesterol and an increased risk of getting heart disease. A food may have no cholesterol, but if it's high in saturated fat, the chemical interactions triggered by the fat that enters the body can make cholesterol levels soar.

In general, those who want to reduce their cholesterol levels should cut back on high-cholesterol foods *and* on foods high in saturated fats. The worst types of fats for increasing cholesterol include butter fat and the so-called tropical fats, such as palm and coconut oil. Some recent studies have suggested that polyunsaturated fats may also raise cholesterol levels.

My recommendation, which conforms to guidelines established by the American Heart Association, is to keep the total consumption of calories involving fats at a level less than 30 percent of your total daily calorie consumption. That 30 percent of total fats should be divided this way:

• One-third saturated fats. These are found in animal foods like beef and lamb; whole milk dairy products; butter; "hydrogenated" foods prepared through commercial processing; and certain vegetable oils like palm oil, coconut oil, and cocoa butter.

• One-third polyunsaturated fats. These are vegetable fats, such as corn oil.

• One-third monounsaturated fats. Olive oil is a prime example of this fat.

Those with cholesterol levels above 240 mg/dl may want to consume 20 percent of their calories as fat, or even less. Those on this type of very low fat diet should continue to observe the proportions of one-third saturated, one-third polyunsaturated, and one-third monounsaturated fats.

High-fiber menus fit nicely into a low-fat, low-cholesterol diet. Remember: The more high-fiber foods you eat, the less high-fat and high-cholesterol foods you'll eat—*automatically!* Through the operation of the substitution principle, there simply won't be room in your stomach for many of the bad foods.

Another note on cholesterol-lowering diets: If you're trying to reduce your cholesterol through a low-fat, low-cholesterol regimen, you'll most likely find that diet will have much more of an impact at the higher levels of cholesterol than at the lower levels.

Many patients whose cholesterol is in the high 200s, for instance, find that they can achieve significant decreases simply by consuming about 30 percent of their total calories as fat. A major reason for this phenomenon is that those with high cholesterol levels are also on a high-fat diet. Consequently, they can often achieve dramatic plunges in their blood tests simply by cutting out a few of the worst foods they're eating.

One woman with a cholesterol level of 280 mg/dl dropped her reading to 235 in a matter of a few weeks on such a diet. She cut back mainly on creamy, high-fat ice cream, two eggs a day, and the fried foods she ate regularly. A man in a similar situation began at 270 mg/dl and went down to 225 on a 30 percent fat diet.

These two people stayed at those levels on their moderate, 30 percent diets. To achieve further reductions, they had to eat a far lower percentage of fats, in the range of 20 to 25 percent of their total calories.

The woman finally got down to a cholesterol level of 165 on a diet involving 20 percent of her calories as fat, but she couldn't seem to go any lower. Further reductions would have required a *very* low fat program, say, 15 percent or lower, and she wasn't willing to make the sacrifice. (In fact, further decreases weren't necessary. Remember: Those whose total cholesterol levels are below 200 are statistically at relatively low risk of developing heart disease.)

The man reached a low plateau of 180. At that point, he decided to go on a near-vegetarian diet, which took him down to 160. He probably could have made it to our baseline range of 120 to 150 mg/dl if he had lost some excess body fat, which can also raise the level of blood cholesterol. But like the woman, he chose to maintain the dietary program that had already greatly reduced his risk of heart disease.

In general, these two people represent an important principle of the impact of diet on blood cholesterol: The higher your cholesterol, the more impact you can expect from dietary restrictions of cholesterol and fats. The lower your cholesterol, the less impact you can expect from diet.

HOW CHOLESTEROL TRAVELS
IN THE BLOODSTREAM

One way I like to describe the problems with dietary cholesterol is to use an image of boats in the bloodstream. Although this concept has been used elsewhere, I employ a little different twist by tying in the idea of an oil spill. Here's the way it works:

Assume that you have a large number of small boats carrying fat back and forth in your blood. These boats, which come in two different sizes, are made of protein and are called lipoproteins. Because fat and blood (which is largely water) don't mix, it would be impossible for the fat to move around by itself to its proper destination, so these special boats are necessary for transport.

The big boats carry cholesterol from the liver to the body's cells tied to a special type of protein—low-density lipoprotein (LDL). As I noted earlier, LDL cholesterol is what is commonly called "bad" cholesterol. Yet the cholesterol carried by LDL is essential to the growth and development of the body's cells. LDL has received bad press because of what can happen if there's an "oil spill" in the bloodstream that isn't cleaned up.

What happens is this: The LDL boats move to the various cells, and much of the LDL cholesterol is used constructively in cell building and repair. Sometimes, though, excess LDL cholesterol spills out into the bloodstream, either because there is too much LDL in the first place (often because of too much cholesterol or fat in the diet), or because the receptors on the cells don't work properly.

When an LDL cholesterol spill occurs, a cholesterol-containing plaque may be formed in the wall of an artery. This obstruction can block the flow of blood and cause a heart attack or stroke.

One of the small boats I referred to earlier may come along and clean up the oil spill. These boats are high-density lipoprotein (HDL), and the cholesterol they carry is often referred to as "good" cholesterol. But while scientists know that high levels of HDL cholesterol are associated with a low incidence of heart disease (and atherosclerosis), they don't know exactly why.

The best theory seems to be that the HDL cholesterol removes cholesterol from plaque in blood vessels and carries it back to the liver. There, some of the cholesterol is eliminated from the body through the gallbladder as bile, which enters the intestinal tract.

Bile is extremely rich in cholesterol, and much of it is stored in the gallbladder before excretion. If something goes wrong with the elimination process, gallstones may develop. Various tests have revealed that gallstones are about 90 percent cholesterol.

In any event, the liver transfers some of the waste cholesterol into the duct leading to the gallbladder, and some goes directly out into the small intestine. The rest of the cholesterol and bile moves into the gallbladder for storage. Finally, the gallbladder bile containing the cholesterol heads back down a duct leading to the small intestine, and from there the waste materials are eliminated from the body.

Unfortunately, the waste removal process doesn't work perfectly. When the cholesterol-containing bile, which comes from both the liver and the gallbladder, pours into the small intestine, some of it goes out of the body through the bowel tract. But some recirculates back into the body through the walls of the small intestine, just like foods and other nutrients. As this recirculating bile goes back into the body, so does the cholesterol.

It's at this point that fiber, which enters the body as part of our food supply, can perform an important additional service: the removal of excess cholesterol.

HOW SOLUBLE FIBER WORKS

You'll recall that I have referred to two main types of fiber: insoluble and soluble. Insoluble fiber will be a primary subject in later chapters. For now, we'll focus on soluble fiber because that's the type that helps to get rid of excess cholesterol in the gastrointestinal tract.

As you already know, soluble fiber, unlike the insoluble variety, doesn't trap water. Instead, as the name implies, it dissolves in water and does its work on the molecular level.

Foods containing cholesterol-reducing soluble fiber include oatmeal, oat bran, dried beans, peas, lentils, and other legumes. These foods tend to be high in substances called lignins and gums, which act to bind the cholesterol. Also, fruits such as apples and strawberries are high in pectin, which has been associated with a reduction of cholesterol.

To understand how soluble fiber works in your body through these foods, let's return to the small intestine. The soluble fiber taken in as food moves through the stomach into the duodenum, the upper part of the small intestine. There, the fiber mixes with the rest of the food and with the bile that has emptied into the small intestine from the liver and gallbladder.

The current theory about how the fiber operates may be summarized this way: The molecular components of the soluble fiber act to tie up or bind the cholesterol that they encounter in the small intestine. In effect, the fiber acts as a kind of chemical net that is drawn so tight that the cholesterol can't escape its clutches. Then, the bound-up cholesterol moves down through the intestinal tract and out of the body, rather than recirculating back into the body. In this way, soluble fiber can help reduce total cholesterol in the bloodstream.

There are some potential drawbacks with soluble fiber, however. As you might expect, the chemical net of this food doesn't just catch excess cholesterol; it also may snag other nutrients that the body really needs. In particular, soluble fiber may reduce the body's supplies of zinc, calcium, and iron.

Clearly, any truly healthy diet must take into account the needs of the individual for *all* nutrients, not just cholesterol. For example, a 60-year-old woman who is suffering from osteoporosis (a condition in which bones become porous) should probably not overload her diet with soluble fiber. If she does, she may lose too much calcium.

I'll deal with the possible dangers of fiber in a later chapter. For now, just keep in mind that if all other nutrients in a person's body are in balance and there is a need for cholesterol reduction, soluble fiber is probably the most natural and safest way to go.

Finally, I want to mention a recent controversy that deals with the impact of the soluble-fiber food oat bran on cholesterol.

In a study reported in January 1990 in *The New England Journal of Medicine*, researchers in Boston found that eating *either* oat bran *or* a low-fiber refined wheat product resulted in similar 7.5 percent reductions in serum cholesterol. The investigators said that the decrease occurred because all the participants in the study ate much less fat and cholesterol after they added the extra oat bran or low-fiber wheat. They concluded that the low-fiber food did as much as the high-fiber oat bran to reduce the level of cholesterol.

But keep in mind the following:

• A substitution effect seems to be in operation here. Substituting a low-fat, low-cholesterol food of any type for high-fat, high-cholesterol foods will lower blood cholesterol levels.

• Many other studies have demonstrated an independent, cholesterol-lowering action on blood cholesterol when soluble-fiber foods like oat bran are added to the diet. So I don't think that the Boston study, which involved only twenty participants, should be interpreted as overturning those studies.

• The Boston results seem to confirm previous studies showing that while soluble fiber reduces "bad" LDL, it doesn't affect "good" HDL cholesterol; this beneficial effect wasn't evident from the low-fiber foods.

The current scientific understanding of soluble fiber on cholesterol may be summed up this way:

1. Soluble fiber helps lower cholesterol in the blood by acting as a substitute for high-fat, high-cholesterol foods that raise serum cholesterol.

2. Soluble fiber apparently has some independent chemical impact on the excess cholesterol it encounters in the small intestine. Specifically, it seems to bind or tie up the extra cholesterol, thus preventing it from recirculating back into the body.

A SOLUBLE-FIBER SOLUTION TO DESIGNING YOUR DIET

Although I'll be presenting a comprehensive food program in Chapters 8 through 10, here are some sample foods that many patients have used to emphasize soluble fiber and lower their cholesterol levels. These are *not* complete, nutritionally balanced menus, so don't use them as such! Rather, they indicate some soluble-fiber, cholesterol-lowering foods you can fit into your diet.

Breakfast: Oatmeal or oat bran cereal, topped with strawberries
Lunch: A whole orange; lentil soup
Afternoon snack: Apple with skin
Supper: Dried beans, peas, or other legumes; half a cup of raspberries

The lowering of cholesterol and the reduction of the risk of heart disease is only the beginning of the fiber story. Next, we'll explore how fiber can function as an effective strategy for countering the threat of cancer.

3

A Counter to Cancer

It amazes me how fiber can help overcome so many of our major health problems.

We've already seen how fiber can combat heart disease, which is the leading killer among all illnesses in our society. Now, as we turn to the second worst killer—cancer—we find fiber once again playing a major preventive role.

Various studies have offered evidence that a diet high in fiber can lower your risk for

- Colon cancer
- Breast cancer
- Stomach cancer
- Various other cancers, such as endometrial, ovarian, and oral

How is it possible for this essentially simple, unglamorous food group to do so much for our health? While the explanation for the anti-cancer action of fiber isn't completely clear, recent studies have removed some of the mystery and now present us with a fairly comprehensive picture of how fiber works to counter cancer.

A COLON CURE-ALL?

A common form of cancer in the United States is cancer of the large intestine, or the colon. This disease, which strikes men and women almost equally, accounts for about one-seventh of all cancers and 60,000 deaths annually.

Yet cancer of the colon isn't inevitable. In fact, the incidence of this disease is relatively low, and in some cases practically nonexistent, in parts of Africa, India, and rural Finland. These societies have something in common: the low rates of colon cancer correlate directly with a high intake of fiber.

Of course, diet isn't the only answer to the colon problem. Early detection of malignancies is also a crucial part of a preventive program. A simple procedure that could dramatically cut the incidence of deaths from colon cancer would be for adults over age 50 to have annual examinations of the colon.

But even before considering this step, we should take a cue from the Africans, Indians, and Finns and make a firmer commitment to fiber. Specifically, there are four basic ingredients that various studies suggest should be part of any effective nutritional action plan against colon cancer.

Ingredient #1:

Include a significant proportion of high-fiber foods in your diet.

Exactly what kind of fiber is best for the prevention of

colon cancer? Answer: The main focus should be on insoluble fiber—although it's important to include soluble fiber as well. (For a list of foods high in soluble and insoluble fiber, see the charts in Chapter 8.)

Lest I seem hopelessly equivocal, let me explain my response by focusing on the intestinal tract of a 52-year-old man named Larry, who happens to be following The Fiber Prescription.

One part of Larry's diet includes insoluble fiber, such as wheat bran. He gets plenty of this substance by eating a hefty bowl of a concentrated wheat bran cereal every morning.

When the insoluble fiber in the cereal reaches Larry's intestines, it softens the stool, decreases the pressure and irritation against the intestinal walls, and reduces the "transit time" of the food and waste through the gastrointestinal tract. By some estimates, it may take only half as long for food to move through the body when fibers are streamlining the transport system. It's been said that eating plenty of insoluble fiber every day is like taking an express train rather than a local to work every morning!

The main advantage of putting your food on such an express train is that there is less time for potentially harmful elements, including carcinogens (cancer producers), to be in contact with the stomach or intestine walls. Less exposure to such dangerous influences means a lower risk of colon cancer.

A second benefit of Larry's diet is that he consumes plenty of soluble fiber, such as wheat bran, corn bran, and dried beans. Scientists believe that soluble fibers trap bile acids, which contain cancer-triggering substances. This chemical-trapping action prevents the bile acids from coming into contact with the gastrointestinal wall. As a result, the chances are reduced that the colon will develop cancer.

Ingredient #2:

Focus on "anti-cancer" vegetables and fruits.

A high-fiber diet will naturally include more vegetables and fruits. But the advantage of these foods extends beyond their fiber content to other cancer-combating nutrients.

For example, some recent research has suggested that vitamin A and beta carotene, which is a precursor to vitamin A, may be protective against cancer of the colon. Vegetables with beta carotene include carrots, kale, lettuce, collards, and broccoli.

Other research indicates that foods containing vitamin C, such as oranges and various other citrus fruits, may also afford protection.

Finally, certain kinds of vegetables known as the "cruciferous" type have been independently associated with lower colon cancer rates. This term, which means "cross," is appropriate because a cross is visible when you split these vegetables down the middle. They include cabbage, cauliflower, brussels sprouts, and broccoli.

Exactly how or why these vegetables or vitamins may be protective against colon cancer isn't known. But preliminary studies indicate that those who eat plenty of these nutrients characteristically suffer a lower incidence of the disease.

Ingredient #3:

Keep your intake of fats low.

Many studies show that a low-fat diet is associated with reduced rates of colon cancer. One theory is that animal fats spread more carcinogenic elements than other foods, especially during the process of breaking the fat down for digestion in the intestines. In contrast, fiber-containing foods release fewer carcinogenic substances when they are fermented during the digestive process.

How about specific guidelines? As I said in the previous chapter, for most people the goal should be to limit consumption of calories derived from fat to no more than 30 percent of total daily calories. Of that 30 percent, no more than one-third should be saturated fat (e.g., bacon fat), one-third monounsaturated fat (e.g., olive oil), and one-third polyunsaturated fat (e.g., corn oil).

And remember, those who consume more fiber *automatically* tend to eat less fat. Larry gained protection because the extra grains, vegetables, and fruits he takes in just don't leave much room for high-fat dishes.

Ingredient #4:

Limit daily calorie intake to *only what you need.*

Taking in too many calories every day can actually increase your risk of colon cancer. I'm the author of a theory on this subject, which involves the following line of reasoning:

The risk for cancer in any organ, such as the colon, depends to some extent on the rate at which the cells in that organ are dividing. The faster the organ's cells divide, the more likely it is that the organ will be afflicted with cancer.

The reason that an organ with a high turnover of cells is more vulnerable to cancer is that cancer-producing substances become operative as the cells are dividing. Conversely, there is less danger to the organ when the cells are "resting," between their division times.

Furthermore, a carcinogen moving through the colon slowly because of a low-fiber diet will be even more likely to attack an intestinal wall. The reason: Lower movement of the carcinogen increases the odds that it will still be in the colon when cells divide.

What determines the rate of cell division? There are two main factors: (1) the number of calories the person eats and (2) the person's age. As more calories are consumed, the rate of cell division increases. Also, as the organ ages, the rate of cell division increases. The opposite is also true: Fewer calories and a younger age are each associated with a slower rate of cell division.

A related factor that may increase the risk of colon cancer is the absolute number of cells in the organ—a consideration that has intriguing implications for the impact of human height and body size.

Some scientific investigations show that tall people have a higher incidence of colon cancer than shorter people. If you break the population into eight groups (octiles) according to height, you find a twofold increase in the incidence of colon cancer when comparing the highest and the lowest octiles.

What practical conclusions can we reach from all this evidence? Here are three points that may help you lower your risk of colon cancer:

1. Limit the calories you eat each day to what's absolutely necessary to maintain an ideal weight. Any excess will raise your risk of cancer.

2. Those who are taller or larger are probably at higher risk for colon cancer than shorter, smaller people. So it's important for the giants or near-giants among us to be particularly diligent in pursuing an anti-cancer regimen.

3. Those who are older are also at higher risk for colon cancer. This means that as we age, increasing our intake of fiber becomes even more essential.

CAN FIBER FIGHT BREAST CANCER?

Although most of the well-known studies focus on the benefits of a high-fiber diet in warding off colon cancer, there are also some intriguing findings about the impact of fiber on breast cancer.

At least two studies have concluded that a high-fiber diet is associated with a lower incidence of breast cancer. In a 1982 report in *The Lancet,* researchers found that the excretion of lignans, a fiber-based substance taken in through diet, was lower in women with breast cancer than in women without cancer.

A similar result emerged in a 1986 investigation published in the *Journal of the National Cancer Institute.* Researchers found that there was an increased risk of breast cancer in women under the age of 50 when they ate diets low in fiber and high in animal fats and protein.

How can a high-fiber diet help to prevent breast cancer? It's hard to arrive at firm conclusions about the precise impact of fiber because of the possible influence of such independent factors as family history in raising the risk for breast cancer. But here is the outline of an explanation that has been offered about how fiber may be involved:

• With a high-fat, low-fiber (and generally low-carbohydrate) diet, human beings tend to reach their full growth potential *and,* in the process, put on extra body fat.

• A woman having higher body fat may experience earlier menarche (the onset of menstruation) and later menopause, with the result that she has a longer exposure to high levels of the female hormone estrogen.

• Exposure to estrogen in the blood has been associated with a higher incidence of breast cancer.

Conversely, Asian women and vegetarians, who are both at low risk for breast cancer, tend to have less estrogen in their blood. Rather, they excrete this hormone in their stool—probably because of their high-fiber, low-fat diets.

Although the final word isn't in yet, the main message in these preliminary findings is that a high-fiber, low-fat diet should be an essential part of any program to combat breast cancer.

More than a quarter of all new cancers each year that strike women in the United States are cancers of the breast. Furthermore, nearly one-tenth of all American women will develop breast cancer during their lifetimes, and about 40,000 die from this disease annually. In light of the magnitude of this threat, it seems that a fiber-focused meal plan is the only nutrition program that makes sense.

WHAT OTHER CANCERS MAY BE COUNTERED BY FIBER?

Only limited studies have been done showing the impact of a high-fiber diet on other types of cancers. Still, the outlook is promising for those that have been investigated.

Stomach cancer has been associated with several definite risk factors, including a high consumption of pickled and salted fish and other high-salt foods. Also, the incidence of this type of cancer is higher in areas where the intake of nitrates in the food is not balanced by the consumption of adequate amounts of vitamin C, vitamin E, and various antioxidants in the food. (Antioxidants, such as vitamins C, E, and A, interfere with the ability of a carcinogen to damage a cell.)

Stomach cancer rates are lower among people whose diets are characterized by a relatively high intake of vitamin C, vitamin E, and other antioxidants and, in general, a high-fiber diet. A high-fiber diet has been related to lower rates of stomach cancer in part because of the substitution effect. That is, the consumption of extra high-fiber foods (and especially those that have not been artificially salted) leaves less room for "bad" foods, such as those that have been pickled or have a high salt content.

In a study conducted in Canada in 1985, researchers found a strong protective effect against stomach cancer among those who consumed high amounts of dietary fiber, including such foods as soybeans, fruits, vegetables, seeds, and nuts. The investigation also concluded that the risk was lower for those who consumed bran cereals. These results confirmed an earlier report from Israel that a decreased risk of stomach cancer is linked to a high-fiber diet.

What are the practical implications of these findings for your diet? In brief, a lower risk of stomach cancer will be associated with a diet including

- Both insoluble and soluble fibers
- Wheat bran and oat bran cereals
- Plenty of vitamin C, which is found in such fruits as oranges, grapefruit, lemons, tangerines, cantaloupe, and strawberries
- Vitamin E sources, such as wheat germ, stone-ground whole wheat flour, cucumbers, and soybean oil

• An avoidance of pickled foods or items otherwise high in salt content

Promising preliminary studies indicate that a high-fiber diet is associated with a lower risk of cancer of the ovaries and cancer of the endometrial lining in the uterus. In addition, cancers of the throat and mouth have been found lower among those on a high-fiber diet, according to a 1988 report in the *Journal of the National Cancer Institute.*

Although these studies have yet to be corroborated, the outlook is more optimistic than originally expected. Clearly, a commitment to fiber is advisable for those who want to maximize their protection against the various forms of the second greatest killer disease that now threatens us.

INSOLUBLE FIBER AT MEALTIMES

Use the following foods as a checklist to be sure you're getting adequate insoluble fiber in your diet—or draw up your own list.

Again, these listings are *not* intended to be a substitute for a complete day's meals. For a properly balanced meal plan, see Chapter 9.

Breakfast: Wheat bran cereal, topped with orange slices
Lunch: Carrots, broccoli
Snack: Pear with skin, wheat bran muffins
Supper: Brussels sprouts, cauliflower, cabbage, lettuce, whole wheat pasta, whole meal bread

With this information on cancer in mind, let's consider some other ways that fiber can be a protective cloak for the colon.

4

A Protective Cloak for the Colon:

Fiber as a Defense Against Constipation and Diverticulitis

Timothy, who suffered from chronic constipation, averaged only two bowel movements a week.

For some people, two movements a week might be enough because the definition of constipation is rather flexible. In general, this condition is described as infrequent, difficult bowel movements. If a person has two or three easy movements a week, he or she may not be considered constipated. On the other hand, most people should have more frequent bowel movements and should experience no strain or pain.

Timothy experimented with various nonprescriptive laxatives, and for several months these medications kept him regular. But before long, as his body adjusted to the drugs, the constipation returned. To Timothy's consternation, he also began to experience intermittent bouts of diarrhea.

Fortunately, Timothy decided the do-it-yourself approach to his problem wasn't working. He consulted with a physician and a qualified nutritionist who had plenty of experience treating constipation. As a result of their advice, he embarked on a high-fiber diet, with an emphasis on insoluble fibers. Almost immediately the natural ability of his intestines to move waste materials through his intestinal tract improved. Within a few weeks, he was back to normal—with regular, easy bowel movements and no need to rely on drugs.

THE ULTIMATE ALL-NATURAL LAXATIVE

As I said at the beginning of this book, most people don't need laxatives to correct constipation. The best response is to change the diet. Specifically, those with constipation should increase their daily fiber and liquid consumption.

Why is fiber so important in combating constipation? In a nutshell, this food softens waste matter in the small and large intestines by promoting the accumulation of water in the stool. As a result, the pressure inside the digestive tract, especially in the large intestine (the colon), decreases. The "transit time" for movement of the waste material then speeds up, and the softened stool can be expelled quickly from the body.

This explanation just scratches the surface. Much more needs to be said about the causes and possible cures of constipation.

THE CAUSES OF CONSTIPATION

First of all, it's important to determine whether or not you really are constipated. Answer the following questions:

• Do you have fewer than two bowel movements a week?

• Do you have trouble passing stools? That is, do you find you must strain, and that the stools are typically small and hard?

• Do you experience pain during bowel movements?

• Is there sometimes blood in your stool after a movement?

• Do you have hemorrhoids?

• Have you experienced increased problems with constipation since becoming pregnant?

Any of these symptoms may indicate the presence of constipation *if* they occur regularly. An occasional problem of this sort is nothing to worry about, however.

Also, if you are well into middle age—say, in your late fifties or older—or if you're pregnant, it's important to pay particular attention to signs of increased constipation. These two categories of people are especially vulnerable.

If you determine you are constipated, there are several common, correctable causes that may underlie the problem. These include a bad diet, use or misuse of certain medications, a lack of exercise, and a failure to observe sound principles of regularity.

Cause #1: Bad Diet.

Constipation may result from the consumption of too many foods that contain large amounts of animal fat, such as meats and whole milk dairy products. Also, fatty, sweet foods like high-calorie desserts may have the same effect.

One of the main problems with this kind of diet is that "bad" foods (e.g., those high in fat) are substituted for "good" ones, such as those high in fiber. A focus on bran cereals, whole-grain breads and pasta, vegetables, and fruits will provide the high fiber necessary to move waste matter easily through the intestinal tract.

How exactly does fiber help prevent constipation?

The mechanism is fairly simple. Food, including fiber, can only be broken down to a limited extent in the stomach. When the food leaves the stomach and enters the small intestine, the breakdown of both soluble and insoluble fiber, along with other foods, continues. In effect, the fiber is "chopped up" by the acids and enzymes in the long, narrow small intestine.

You'll recall that at this stage of digestion, soluble fiber (such as oat bran) binds excess cholesterol so that it can move out of the body as waste, rather than back into the body and bloodstream.

The waste matter, including fiber, then moves from the small intestine to the large intestine (the colon). There, the insoluble fiber, which is found in such foods as wheat bran cereals and various vegetables, really goes to work.

In the colon, bacteria attack the fiber and begin a fermentation process, which leads to the release of gases. Until the body gets used to a high-fiber diet, this flatulence can make a person feel rather uncomfortable. (But take heart—the gas does decrease as the body adjusts.)

At this stage, however, the gas production is only a temporary, mildly unpleasant by-product of a much more significant set of events. The most important function of the insoluble fiber is to absorb water in the large intestine and thus increase the size and softness of the stool. The cellulose in insoluble fiber cannot be digested, but it can take in water, somewhat like a sponge. This process helps prevent constipation.

Without sufficient fiber, the water is reabsorbed into the body through the walls of the colon, and the stool becomes hard and small. The longer the waste stays in the colon—i.e., the longer its "transit time" in the intestinal tract—the harder it becomes. This process of hardening of the stool is the source of constipation.

The Fluid Factor. Whenever I talk about the importance of diet, I always try to include some reference to liquids—especially where constipation is concerned.

One of the essential ingredients in developing a soft, fast-moving stool is *water*. Granted, there must be sufficient fiber to absorb the water, but without enough liquids in your system, the action of the fiber will be limited.

The usual, well-worn rule says to drink eight 8-ounce glasses of water, or the equivalent in fruit juices, every day. That's a good goal to shoot for, but don't worry if you don't quite make it. If you eat plenty of fruits and other foods that contain large amounts of water, you'll be able to meet your quota.

Probably the best way to ensure that you'll have enough fluids is to drink at least one 8-ounce glass of water at every meal, drink an 8-ounce glass of fruit juice at breakfast and at one other time during the day, and eat plenty of fruit. Then, any other consumption of water during the day will probably provide you with enough to cover your basic needs.

Caution: In calculating your liquid consumption, *don't* include alcoholic drinks, which tend to dehydrate the body. Also, in your calculation omit milk products, which are certainly important for calcium and other nutrients but may cause constipation in some people.

How About Fiber Extracts? The use of insoluble fiber extracts, such as Metamucil, can trigger a fiber action to prevent constipation. Usually, though, it's best to take the natural approach—that is, to change your diet so that fiber comes in through daily food intake. The reason for my bias is that high-fiber foods contain important nutrients, including various vitamins and minerals, that aren't in the supplements. Changing the basic diet through high-fiber meals always multiplies the health benefits.

Constipation and Pregnancy. Pregnant women often complain about constipation, and there are two possible reasons for the problem. One is simply the pressure of the developing fetus on the intestinal tract. As the growing baby increases in size and weight, there is less room in the abdominal area for other organs, such as the large intestine. This means that food waste must move through a narrower opening, and difficulty in bowel movements may result.

There's a tendency for pregnant women to switch to foods outside their normal dietary range as a result of unusual cravings. These nutritional shifts may trigger bowel problems. Also, the hormonal changes that occur during pregnancy may affect the digestive process in some women and make the movement of food and waste through the gastrointestinal tract more sluggish.

In a 1985 report in *Human Nutrition*, researchers A. S. Anderson and M. J. Whichelow studied forty women who complained of constipation during the third trimester of pregnancy. The women were divided into three groups, with the following changes in their diets:

Group A increased their average intake of fiber by 7.2 grams a day in the form of a corn-based biscuit. Group B increased their fiber by 9.1 grams a day through the consumption of wheat bran. Group C continued without medical intervention, and in fact decreased their fiber intake by 3.5 grams a day.

The results of the study showed that the dietary changes were accompanied by a change to a softer stool and an increase in the number of bowel movements in Groups A and B, which had increased their fiber intake. There were no changes in the number of bowel movements or the stool consistency in the third group.

The message for pregnant women in such studies is clear: Embark on a full-fiber meal plan!

Cause #2: Use or Misuse of Medications.

Sometimes certain medications may cause constipation as a side effect. These include diuretics for high blood pressure, medications used to fight Parkinson's disease, antacids with calcium or aluminum ingredients, some antidepressant drugs, and antihistamines.

If your problem stems from such medications, your doctor may be able to reduce the dosages or prescribe alternate drugs that don't cause constipation.

A more insidious link of drugs to constipation is the misuse of laxatives, as happened with Timothy in the earlier example. Reports from the National Institute on Aging and elsewhere have estimated that Americans spend $250 million a year on over-the-counter laxatives.

The problem with these drugs is that while they may help overcome constipation at first, they can become habit-forming. Furthermore, the natural waste-handling mechanisms of the body tend to "shut down" as heavier reliance is placed on these substances. Finally, the drugs themselves become less effective, and constipation or even diarrhea may occur.

Regular use of enemas or other artificial devices may have a similar effect in causing the natural bowel mechanism to stop functioning properly.

Other problems that may occur with persistent use of laxatives include the disruption of the flow of needed nutrients into the body. For example, the use of mineral oil may interfere with the absorption of vitamins A, D, E, and K into the blood and tissues.

My advice: Stay away from over-the-counter laxatives completely unless your doctor advises otherwise. As an alternative, increase the amount of fiber in your diet.

Cause #3: Lack of Exercise.

It's common for those who are confined to bed or who are inactive during an extended illness or accident to develop constipation. For that matter, a sedentary lifestyle among otherwise healthy people may aggravate bowel problems.

The reason exercise is so important isn't entirely clear. But most explanations include an emphasis on the importance of keeping the body's muscles, circulatory system, and various organs in regular use.

A failure to use any part of our complex physical systems will inevitably lead to malfunctions in those systems—and one of the most common signals of disuse is problems in the digestive tract. Consequently, any high-fiber diet program should be supplemented by a reasonable amount of exercise, including regular walking and other physical activity.

Cause #4: Failure to Observe Sound Principles of Regularity.

Although this point may seem too obvious to mention, many physicians include it at the top of their checklist for patients who complain of constipation.

The question put to the patient by the physician may be rather blunt: "Do you go *directly* to the toilet when you feel it's time?" Often, the honest answer is no.

Many people may fail to respond because they are busy with other interests or responsibilities. Others are too lazy and postpone getting up for a few minutes. Unfortunately, the signal may not return, and the delay may cause the stool to harden, thus leading to constipation.

Responding when the time is right can be particularly important for older people or pregnant women, who are more prone as groups to constipation.

The Hemorrhoid Connection. One of the unpleasant byproducts of constipation may be the development of hemorrhoids. These are blood vessels surrounding the anus and rectum that become weak and enlarged, often because of the straining that accompanies constipation.

If untreated, these balloonlike protrusions may grow larger, become inflamed, and even begin to bleed. In addition to various creams that are effective in soothing and reducing the size of the hemorrhoids, a change to a high-fiber diet will help ease the strain and pain associated with constipation.

A NATURAL CURE FOR CONSTIPATION

To relieve constipation, the best diet will include all types of high-fiber foods, with an emphasis on those that include insoluble fiber, including cellulose and hemicellulose.

The best foods to soften and enlarge the stool are wheat bran muffins and cereals high in wheat bran. Many people find that oat bran muffins and other oat products are helpful. In addition, fresh vegetables and fruits, such as broccoli, carrots, apples, prunes, and pears, will combat constipation.

How much of these high-fiber foods should you eat to overcome constipation? The answer is always a matter of individual response, but remember: The average American takes in an average of 10 to 15 grams of fiber a day. In contrast, as you already know, I recommend a minimum of 20 to 30 grams. That means *at least* one large bowl of wheat bran cereal, four or five vegetables, and two or three pieces of fruit each day, in addition to other foods normally consumed.

The effect of such a diet on constipation can be extremely beneficial, as the following medical studies suggest:

• In a 1985 study on the impact of diet on constipation, researcher J. C. Valle-Jones had fifty elderly patients add oat bran meal biscuits twice daily to their diets. The treatment caused a marked improvement in bowel frequency, greater stool consistency, and reduction in pain on defecation. No patients complained of side effects.

• In a 1984 report on constipation in the aged, researcher J. W. Merkus noted that although about 50 percent of the elderly use laxatives, the main cause of their constipation is a lack of dietary fiber. He also found that constipation among the elderly may have dangerous complications, such as acute mental confusion, retention of urine, urinary incontinence, and impacting of fecal matter. Because laxatives may have harmful side effects, Merkus recommended increasing fiber in daily menus.

• Researcher V. van den Brandt-Gradel reported in a 1984 study that a high-fiber diet, accompanied by reduced straining during bowel movements, caused a significant improvement in rectal ulcers. In fifteen patients, ulcer symptoms disappeared completely and sores were healed in less than eleven months after the beginning of the high-fiber regimen.

Of course, switching to a high-fiber diet may not solve the problem of constipation for everyone. Some people may have blockages caused by intestinal obstructions or by nerve or muscle inadequacy in the digestive system. In such cases, other medical or surgical steps will have to be taken. But for most of us, a high-fiber diet, along with adequate intake of fluids and regular exercise, should be adequate to eliminate the scourge of constipation.

As we've seen in our discussions of cancer and constipation, fast transit time in the intestinal tract is a major plus for good health. The same holds true for another common problem that plagues many older people—the weakening and "outpouching" of the colon wall that begins as diverticulosis and may well turn into the more serious condition, diverticulitis.

PROTECTION AGAINST DIVERTICULITIS

Ronald, a 61-year-old executive, started to suffer mild pain in the lower left side of his abdomen. He had disregarded this warning signal at first because he assumed that he was just having gas problems.

The pain continued, however, along with a tenderness on the lower left side. Ronald began to run a low-grade fever, experienced frequent diarrhea, and once even noticed blood in his stool.

By this time, Ronald knew something was wrong, so he contacted his doctor. The diagnosis was swift and certain: he had a mild case of diverticulitis, or an inflammation of outpouchings that had developed on the walls of his colon.

How Did Ronald Get Diverticulitis?

Diverticulitis actually begins with a condition known as diverticulosis, the formation of small sacs on the wall of the colon, or large intestine. By conservative estimates, at least 20 percent of people age 60 and older have diverticulosis, and some experts say that the majority of people over 60 are afflicted.

The problem is caused by areas in the wall of the colon that grow weaker and weaker over the years as they are subjected to the constant pressure necessary to propel the food and waste through the intestine. Eventually, this steady pressure creates small outpouchings of the wall of the colon, called diverticuli. Diverticulosis is the condition of having these outpouchings in the colon.

Sometimes, food or other material and bacteria become stuck in one or more diverticuli in the colon, and infection follows. The inflammation and irritation that accompany infection signal the onset of the more serious condition, diverticulitis, and may cause severe pain and fever. Fortunately for Ronald, he saw his doctor before the condition became this serious.

In the worst cases, the pouches may even rupture and trigger highly dangerous peritonitis. Peritonitis, which involves infection of the abdominal lining, can present much the same threat to health or even life as a ruptured appendix. In fact, the appendix is a natural, large pouch or diverticulum on the right side of the colon, and appendicitis is a close relative of diverticulitis.

In more specific and personal terms, here's how Ronald's diverticulitis evolved over the years:

Ronald ate a low-fiber diet most of his life. He concentrated mainly on meats and often said, only half-jokingly, "Vegetables are for women and kids." That mistake contributed to infrequent, hard bowel movements, often only three times a week. The resulting constant, high level of pressure on his colon led to the development of outpouchings (diverticuli), and eventually to diverticulitis.

Ronald's problem was that he had chosen a meal plan that ran counter to the basic needs and functioning of his body. The gastrointestinal tract is a tube, and the muscles in the lining of the tract squeeze and contract to push food from one end to the other. The undulating effect of these steady contractions and relaxations moves the digesting food and debris from the juncture of the stomach and small intestine into the colon, and finally out of the body through the rectum.

Whatever you squeeze, however—whether it's a toothpaste tube or the human intestine—will create resistance against some wall or container. So as the material inside the gastrointestinal tract is squeezed harder, as happened with Ronald's hard stool, pressure increases against the intestinal walls. Not only that, the harder the material is and the more slowly it moves, the harder the squeezing action must be.

As you can probably surmise by now, the pressure that must be exerted against the intestinal wall depends directly on the diet that the person eats. Meals that are low in fiber will result in slower-moving, harder stools and will require more pressure to squeeze them through the tract. In contrast, meals high in fiber will be bulkier, softer, and swifter in movement and will require less pressure.

(A closely related issue is the link between the speed of movement of the stool and appendicitis. A 1985 study in the *Annals of Gynaecology* reported that bowel actions per week were significantly fewer in a group of patients with acute appendicitis than in a group of healthy volunteers. The researcher, E. Arnbjornssen, found support for the idea that the obstruction of the colon around the appendix is a key factor in the development of acute appendicitis.)

A similar process occurs with diverticuli elsewhere in the colon. As this squeezing action continued over the years, Ronald developed a number of outpouchings on his large intestine, probably during his forties or early fifties.

These sacs, which arose in direct response to the high pressure against Ronald's large intestine wall, occurred in areas that were naturally weaker than others. You know, for instance, if you have a balloon with several weak spots, those spots tend to bulge out as the balloon is inflated. That's similar to what happens with diverticuli.

This process resulting in intestinal outpouchings has been confirmed by the use of devices that are inserted into the colon to measure the pressure exerted by the squeezing action of the muscles on the stool. The pressure is always greater when the stool is harder. Also, the pressure against the intestinal wall is greater among those patients with diverticulosis.

The converse is also true: Medical researchers have demonstrated that when a person is put on a high-fiber diet, the stool softens and the pressure in the colon decreases quickly.

Other evidence shows unequivocally that the older you are, the more likely it is that you have diverticuli. The constant pressure against the colon over a period of years or decades eventually causes the weaker areas to bulge out. The lesson for us: A high-fiber diet is important throughout life to prevent the development or enlargement of any outpouchings on the colon. Such a diet becomes even more important the older we get. .

If steps aren't taken to reduce the pressure, the diverticuli will become more pronounced and more likely to trap debris moving through the colon. When food becomes stuck in one of these sacs, a resulting infection will convert diverticulosis to diverticulitis.

This sequence of intestinal events describes what happened to Ronald. But he was lucky. If his condition had gone untreated, other, extremely serious complications might have arisen from his mild diverticulitis. Here are some possible scenarios:

• The infected sacs may begin to bleed. Sometimes bleeding may occur without infection and may clear up quickly. If the bleeding is heavy, however, surgery may be necessary to correct the problem.

• As we saw earlier, an infected sac may burst and infect

the surrounding abdominal lining, thus leading to the dangerous condition known as peritonitis. As with a ruptured appendix, surgery will be necessary in this case.

• Severe, untreated infections may become isolated abscesses in the colon and may cause infection in other parts of the lower body, including the vagina or bladder. Most likely, surgery will be required.

• Continuing infections may cause the walls of the colon to bulge inward. This narrowing of the intestinal pathway may lead to blockages that can be confused with cancer of the colon. Exploratory surgery may be prescribed to ascertain the true nature of the problem.

Obviously, you don't want to confront any of these problems. Fortunately, Ronald didn't have to, either. He saw his doctor in time, and so less serious countermeasures could be taken to correct his illness.

THE PROTECTIVE CLOAK: HOW FIBER HELPED RONALD

The first step in treating Ronald was to fight the infection that had struck his colon. He began taking low dosages of the antibiotic tetracycline. After a couple of days' bedrest, he was feeling much better.

Ronald continued on the medication for about ten days, until the infection had been wiped out completely. At the same time, he switched to a high-fiber diet in an effort to decrease the pressure on his colon and speed up the movement of his stool through the intestinal tract.

Ronald's dietary prescription included at least 30 grams of fiber a day. The foods involved more whole-grain bread and cereals, vegetables, fruits, and wheat and oat bran products than he had been eating previously. His typical daily fiber intake is summarized below. For the sake of simplicity, I've omitted meats and other low-fiber nutrients. This emphasis on fiber is intended both to overcome any tendency toward constipation and to ease the symptoms of diverticulitis.

Breakfast: A popular concentrated wheat bran cereal, topped by a sliced whole banana, strawberries, or a sliced orange

Lunch: A bran muffin; at least two lightly cooked vegetables, such as broccoli or spinach

Snack: An apple with skin and another bran muffin

Dinner: A third bran muffin; another high-fiber vegetable, such as brussels sprouts; a baked potato

These high-fiber additions to Ronald's meals added more than 33 grams of fiber to his diet. The balance of both insoluble- and soluble-fiber foods in his meal plan is consistent with the full-fiber menus and recipes included in this book.

As a result of these changes in his eating, Ronald has begun to have more frequent and easier bowel movements. Just as important, the symptoms of diverticulitis have not returned. Apparently, the reduced pressure in his colon, combined with the faster transit time of food in his gastrointestinal tract, has solved his colon problems.

In addition to providing a protective cloak for the colon, a high-fiber diet has other important benefits. One of the most significant, which increasing numbers of dieters are discovering, is that meals packed with fiber are an ideal prescription for weight loss.

5

A Little-Known Secret for Successful Weight Control

Marcus, an advertising company employee in his late thirties, knew from medical evaluations that he was about twenty pounds above his ideal weight. In addition to being unattractive, the excess weight seemed to be contributing to a couple of health problems.

For one thing, Marcus had been suffering from mild hypertension, with blood pressure measurements averaging 160/95 mm Hg. (Normal blood pressure is below 140/90.) Also, his total cholesterol was 240 mg/dl, when it should have been below 200. These two problems placed Marcus at higher risk for stroke and heart attack, and as his doctor quite correctly pointed out, the extra weight was aggravating the threat to his health.

An examination of Marcus's diet revealed a high-fat, low-fiber diet. His meals emphasized regular helpings of hamburger, lamb, fried chicken, and fried potatoes. At least once a day he had a high-fat dessert, such as cake or pie. Typical snacks included cheddar cheese and crackers before supper and ice cream at bedtime.

Marcus argued that despite the type of food he was eating, he was careful to limit himself to relatively small portions. "And I never go back for seconds," he said. Still, a nutritional analysis showed that on a typical day, 38 percent of the calories he consumed came from fats, 25 percent from protein, and only 37 percent from carbohydrates, including high-fiber foods. The American Heart Association, in contrast, recommends that a maximum of 30 percent of daily calories come from fats, with about 50 percent from carbohydrates and 20 percent from protein.

To maximize Marcus's chances of lowering his weight, as well as his cholesterol and blood pressure levels, his doctor went even further than the AHA: He suggested that Marcus try to consume no more than 20 percent of calories each day from fats, no more than 15 percent from protein, and 65 percent from carbohydrates, including high-fiber dishes.

Note the substitutionary philosophy behind this recommendation. In effect, the doctor was asking Marcus to flip-flop his food plan so as to double his intake of carbohydrates and halve his consumption of fats and protein foods. The carbohydrates—which emphasized high-fiber complex carbohydrates like fresh vegetables, fruits, whole-grain cereals, oat bran muffins, and other bran items—took the place of fatty, high-protein foods like red meat, whole milk dairy products, and heavy desserts.

Marcus followed a particular eating strategy. At his doctor's suggestion, he always tried to eat the high-fiber items first to fill up his stomach and stave off hunger pangs. For example, he began to eat at least one full helping of an extra vegetable at each meal. Also, instead of immediately going for his usual snacks, such as cheese or ice cream, he chose as a substitute a high-fiber fruit, such as a pear or strawberries.

At first, Marcus wasn't enthusiastic about the new meal plan. But after only a week, he found that loading up on the bulky, high-fiber foods left little room for high-fat dishes.

"If you still have room left, go ahead and eat some of the meats and sweets," the doctor had said.

But there wasn't much room. Also, Marcus found that his food preferences began to change. After only about three weeks, he didn't enjoy fatty foods as much as he had in the past. In fact, when he drank some whole milk once by mistake, he discovered that "it seemed oily or slimy. I could actually taste the extra fat, and I didn't like it."

Marcus also increased his level of physical activity in an effort to burn off calories. Specifically, he tried to average about ten miles of fast walking each week.

The results of these relatively mild and palatable changes in diet and lifestyle were dramatic. Marcus lost the extra twenty pounds in only ten weeks, or an average of two pounds a week. Just as important, his blood pressure dropped to the normal range, and his cholesterol hovered around 195.

Although Marcus's doctor had never talked about calories, the weight loss could be attributed mainly to the shift away from fats and toward carbohydrates. In terms of the quantity of the food consumed, Marcus was actually eating more than he had previously. But the calories were considerably less because fat carries more calories per gram than do carbohydrates.

Specifically, there are about 9 calories in every gram of fat consumed, while there are only about 4 calories in every gram of carbohydrate. (There are also 4 calories in every gram of protein.) This means that when Marcus ate 20 grams of fat in a piece of steak, he was taking in 180 calories just from the fat. In contrast, when he consumed 20 grams of carbohydrate in some fruits or vegetables, he was taking in about 80 calories. By substituting high-fiber carbohydrates for fat, he was able to cut his calorie consumption in half, even as he consumed equal amounts of food.

Although Marcus's experience tells us a lot about how a high-fiber diet can overcome obesity, his story is only an introduction to the issue. Let's explore in more depth the definitions, dangers, and causes of obesity—and how you can employ The Fiber Prescription as a way to control your weight.

WHAT IS OBESITY?

Obesity is the physical condition characterized by too much body fat. But trying to evaluate a person's body fat status by measuring height and weight often isn't a very reliable method, even though many insurance companies still use this measure.

The problem is that some people have heavy bones and muscles, while others are light-framed. As a result, certain short people may seem to be obese on height–weight charts, but in fact they may have a very low percent of body fat. Similarly, some light-framed people may appear to be fine on the height–weight listings, but they may really be quite obese because they have a high proportion of body fat.

Because of the difficulty of measuring percent of body fat outside a clinic or laboratory, it's useful to rely on a scientifically tested scale known as a nomogram. Using this scale, you can evaluate your level of obesity fairly well by a concept known as the body mass index (BMI). All you need to know is your weight unclothed and your height barefoot. Then, use the accompanying nomogram to find your BMI.

In general, a person is overweight if his or her BMI is more than 27 to 30 on the nomogram scale. Because there are some variations according to age, however, a more precise listing of desirable body mass indexes also has been included.

Please note: Body Mass Index (BMI) is a method for determining body composition (i.e., the amount of lean body mass and fat) and therefore is valid for both sexes.

If you determine from the nomogram that your body mass index (and weight) are too high, try this maneuver with the straight edge you're using:

Keep the end pointing to your height stationary, but gradually move the other end down until the straight edge cuts through the BMI scale at the range of your desirable weight. Now, look back at the weight scale and see the poundage that the straight edge indicates. This weight will be close to your ideal weight.

WHAT ARE THE DANGERS OF BEING OVERWEIGHT?

You've already been introduced to two of the big dangers of obesity through the story of Marcus. He was beset by high blood pressure (hypertension) and high cholesterol. Hypertension is one of the biggest risk factors associated with stroke.

Increasing levels of overweight have also been linked to increasing risk of non-insulin-dependent diabetes mellitus. In addition, those who are overweight face a higher risk of certain types of cancers, such as those of the gallbladder,

NOMOGRAM TO DETERMINE BODY MASS INDEX

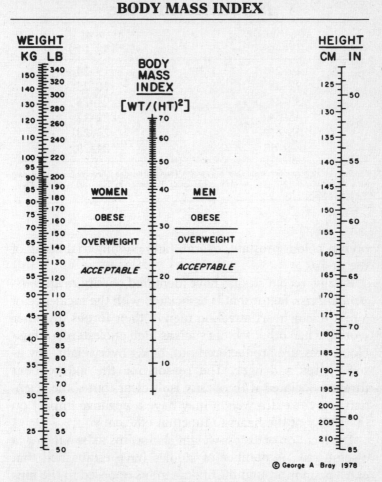

© George A Bray 1978

To use this nomogram, place a ruler or other straight edge between the body weight in kilograms or pounds (without clothes) located on the left-hand column and the height in centimeters or inches (without shoes) located on the right-hand column. The BMI is read from the middle of the scale and is in metric units. Copyright 1978, George A. Bray. Used with permission. Original source of publication: *The International Journal of Obesity.*

DESIRABLE BODY MASS INDEX IN RELATION TO AGE

AGE GROUP (years)	BMI (kg/m²)
19–24	19–24
25–34	20–25
35–44	21–26
45–54	22–27
55–65	23–28
over 65	24–29

Reprinted with permission from *Diet and Health: Implications for Reducing Chronic Disease Risk*, © 1989 by the National Academy of Sciences. Published by National Academy Press, Washington, DC.

breast, colon, prostate, ovaries, and endometrial lining of the uterus.

Finally, recent studies have identified obesity as an *independent* risk factor that is associated with the incidence of a first major heart attack in men in their forties. In other words, when other factors such as high cholesterol or high blood pressure are factored out, being overweight—by itself—poses a danger. The reason for the independent threat associated with obesity isn't clear, but some scientists feel the extra weight may have a negative impact on the ability of the heart to function efficiently.

The location of excess weight also seems to be a factor in disease risk. A number of studies have established that extra pounds around the abdomen, as opposed to the hips or legs, put a person at a greater risk of premature death and of heart disease.

WHAT CAUSES OBESITY?

A great deal has been written recently about the causes of obesity—and the supposed reasons why people who "take it off" can't "keep it off." Despite the confusion and complex argumentation surrounding this subject, the possible sources of the problem are rather simple.

Cause #1: Inherited Tendency to Be Fat. Obesity definitely does run in families. Among other things, studies of twins have established that there is undoubtedly a genetic component in some obesity.

Also, patterns of developing fat on the body may be inherited. For example, Mexican-American children have shown a tendency to develop more fat tissue on the upper body, while those of European extraction are more likely to become fat around the stomach and hips.

A related genetic problem is the way the individual's metabolism handles food.

The way your body consumes calories is reminiscent of the way your car consumes its fuel. A car that burns fuel efficiently uses less gas than a "gas guzzler." Similarly, a person who metabolizes food efficiently burns off relatively few calories—and, as a consequence, has more calories remaining that can be stored as body fat.

In contrast, a person who makes use of food less efficiently will tend to burn up more calories in generating the same amount of energy. As such, he has fewer calories left over that can be stored as fat. Ironically, then, if you want to avoid obesity, it's actually better for the body to operate *less* efficiently!

In some cases, then, genes play a big role in obesity. But

I think an overemphasis on the genetic component has become a cop-out for many people. To be sure, some of us may have trouble keeping off excess weight. But most people can at least control their overweight tendencies by paying close attention to the following two causes, which may be at the root of their problem.

Cause #2: Too Little Exercise. When the intake of fuel in the form of calories is greater than the expenditure of those calories through exercise, excess weight will accumulate.

The accompanying table shows how many calories are used up every minute by various types of activities. As you can see, just walking at a fairly brisk pace of 4.5 miles per hour will use up 180 to 210 calories in a half hour. Furthermore, burning off 3,600 calories more than you take in will take off one pound. So, if you walk enough to burn off 300 extra calories a day, you can take off one pound in just twelve days—just through exercise!

Cause #3: Too Much Food. This cause may seem too obvious to include, but manipulating the diet, after all, is what successful weight reduction is all about for the majority of us.

Only a small number of people have such serious genetic problems that lifestyle changes are ineffective for weight loss. Also, few have the time or inclination to exercise intensely and regularly enough to control their weight only through physical activity. That confronts us with the challenge of dealing with our diets—and The Fiber Prescription can provide one of the most effective and tastiest solutions.

CALORIES USED UP
BY COMMON ACTIVITIES

APPROX. KCAL/MIN.

MOST DEMANDING

Cross-country skiing	5 mph	11–12
Running	7 mph	12–14
Karate		10–13
Bicycling	13 mph	10–12
Basketball (full court)		10–12

MODERATELY DEMANDING

Swimming (crawl, 50 meters/min.)		9–11
Skating (vigorous)		9–10
Handball		9–11
Squash		10–12
Running/jogging	5.5 mph	10–12
Tennis (vigorous singles)		9–10
Downhill skiing with tight turns		8–10
Bicycling	11 mph	7–8
Racquetball		7–10

LESS DEMANDING

Walking	4.5 mph	6–7
Skating (moderately vigorous)		5–7
Tennis (moderately vigorous)		7–8
Canoeing	4 mph	7–8
Badminton (vigorous)		6–8
Folk (square) dancing		6–9

SOURCE: From *Diet and Exercise: Synergism in Health Maintenance*, Philip L. White and Therese Mondeika, eds. Chicago: American Medical Association, 1982, p. 133.

HOW FIBER WORKS AS
A DIET FOOD

Scientific studies have established that high-fiber foods *can* eliminate excess weight. Here are some illustrations from the medical literature:

• A 1984 study reported in the *British Journal of Nutrition* required twenty-one obese people to include in their diets 10 grams of guar gum twice a day every other week over a ten-week period. On alternate weeks, they were asked to substitute similar amounts of wheat bran. During the program, the participants were asked to maintain their regular dietary habits.

The program resulted in "significant" weight reductions, according to the researchers. Specifically, while on the guar-gum-plus-wheat-bran regimen, the patients dropped from an average of 92.5 kilograms in body weight to an average of 85.4 kilograms. They averaged a 0.94 kilogram weekly loss on the guar gum weeks, and a 0.64 kilogram loss on the wheat bran weeks.

In addition to weight reduction, consuming the guar gum, which can be found in oat bran, oat products, and various legumes like dried beans, reduced patients' hunger and lowered total cholesterol.

• A 1988 report in the *Journal of the American Dietetic Association* found that wheat bran supplements didn't affect body weight, but other types of fiber did have a weight-reduction effect.

The studies reviewed in this article were criticized on a number of grounds. Among other things, the studies were short term and involved low doses of fiber. Even with such poorly constructed investigations, however, fiber seemed to work to some extent.

• According to a 1985 article in *Current Medical Research*, there was a significant average weight reduction in fifty elderly patients who ate oat bran meal biscuits twice a day for twelve weeks.

• A 1985 review article in the *Journal of Environmental Pathology, Toxicology, and Oncology* supported the idea that low-fiber foods that cause excess insulin secretion may lead to obesity. In contrast, high-fiber foods that provoke less of an insulin response may help control obesity. The authors noted that high insulin levels are a universal characteristic of obesity and may be a cause of the problem.

To sum up, these and related studies suggest that there are several mechanisms by which fiber can help combat obesity.

First of all, eating relatively large quantities of lower-calorie, high-fiber carbohydrates will fill the stomach and lead to a sense of "being full." In this way, there will be less of a drive to take in fatty foods, which carry more calories per gram of weight.

To give you a better idea of how much fiber is contained in certain popular foods and also the calorie content of those foods, I've included the accompanying chart from the American Dietetic Association.

A second way that fiber combats obesity is by blocking entry to calories. Some studies have shown that doubling or tripling the intake of fiber in the diet can reduce the "digestibility of energy" in the gastrointestinal tract by about 2 percent. In other words, 2 percent fewer calories are absorbed by the body.

Although a 2 percent reduction may not seem like much, this energy loss translates into 50 to 100 calories a day.

DIETARY FIBER AND CALORIES FOR COMMON FOODS

FOOD	FIBER (GM)/ 100 GM*	CALORIES/ 100 GM	SERVING SIZE	FIBER (GM)/ SERVING	CALORIES/ SERVING
BREAKFAST CEREALS					
All-Bran			⅓ c (1 oz)	8.5	71
Bran Buds			⅓ c (1 oz)	7.9	73
Bran Chex			⅔ c (1 oz)	4.6	91
Cheerios-type			1¼ c (1 oz)	1.1	111
Corn Bran			⅔ c (1 oz)	5.4	98
Cracklin' Bran			⅓ c (1 oz)	4.3	108
Crispy Wheats n' Raisins			¾ c (1 oz)	1.3	99
40% Bran-type			¾ c (1 oz)	4.0	93
Frosted Mini Wheats			4 biscuits (1 oz)	2.1	102
Graham Crackos			¾ c (1 oz)	1.7	102
Grape-Nuts			¼ c (1 oz)	1.4	101
Heartland Natural Cereal, plain			¼ c (1 oz)	1.3	123
HoneyBran			⅞ c (1 oz)	3.1	97
Most			⅔ c (1 oz)	3.5	95
Nutri-Grain, barley			¾ c (1 oz)	1.7	106
Nutri-Grain, corn			¾ c (1 oz)	1.8	108
Nutri-Grain, rye			¾ c (1 oz)	1.8	102
Nutri-Grain, wheat			¾ c (1 oz)	1.8	102
100% Bran			½ c (1 oz)	8.4	76
100% Natural Cereal, plain			¼ c (1 oz)	1.0	133
Raisin Bran-type			¾ c (1 oz)	4.0	115

*Dietary fiber values are averages compiled from literature sources.
SOURCE: Adapted from *Journal of the American Dietetic Association*, June 1986, pp. 737–739.

DIETARY FIBER AND CALORIES FOR COMMON FOODS *(continued)*

FOOD	FIBER (GM)/ 100 GM*	CALORIES/ 100 GM	SERVING SIZE	FIBER (GM)/ SERVING	CALORIES/ SERVING
Shredded Wheat			⅔ c (1 oz)	2.6	102
Tasteeos			1¼ c (1 oz)	1.0	111
Total			1 c (1 oz)	2.0	100
Wheat 'n' Raisin Chex			¾ c (1⅓ oz)	2.5	130
Wheat Chex			⅔ c (1⅓ oz)	2.1	104
Wheaties			1 c (1 oz)	2.0	99
oatmeal, regular, quick, and instant, cooked			¾ c (1 oz)	1.6	108
wheat germ			¼ c (2 oz)	3.4	108
Cornflakes			1¼ c (1 oz)	0.3	110
Rice Krispies			1 c (1 oz)	0.1	112
Special K			1⅓ c (1 oz)	0.2	111
Sugar Smacks			¾ c (1 oz)	0.4	106
FRUITS					
apple (w/o skin)			1 med.	2.7	72
apple (w/skin)			1 med.	3.5	81
apricot (fresh)			3 med.	1.8	51
apricot, dried			5 halves	1.4	42
banana			1 med.	2.4	105
blueberries			½ c	2.0	39
cantaloupe			¼ melon	1.0	30
cherries, sweet			10	1.2	49
dates			3	1.9	68
grapefruit			½	1.6	38

71

DIETARY FIBER AND CALORIES FOR COMMON FOODS *(continued)*

FOOD	FIBER (GM)/ 100 GM*	CALORIES/ 100 GM	SERVING SIZE	FIBER (GM)/ SERVING	CALORIES/ SERVING
grapes			20	0.6	30
orange			1	2.6	62
peach (w/skin)			1	1.9	37
peach (w/o skin)			1	1.2	37
pear (w/skin)			½ large	3.1	61
pear (w/o skin)			½ large	2.5	61
pineapple			½ c	1.1	39
plums, damsons			5	0.9	33
prunes			3	3.0	60
raisins			¼ c	3.1	108
raspberries			½ c	3.1	35
strawberries			1 c	3.0	45
watermelon			1 c	0.4	42
juices					
apple			½ c (4 oz)	0.4	56
grapefruit			½ c (4 oz)	0.5	51
grape			½ c (4 oz)	0.6	64
orange			½ c (4 oz)	0.5	56
papaya			½ c (4 oz)	0.8	71
VEGETABLES					
cooked					
asparagus, cut			½ c	1.0	15
beans, string, green			½ c	1.6	16

72

DIETARY FIBER AND CALORIES FOR COMMON FOODS *(continued)*

FOOD	FIBER (GM)/ 100 GM*	CALORIES/ 100 GM	SERVING SIZE	FIBER (GM)/ SERVING	CALORIES/ SERVING
broccoli			½ c	2.2	20
brussels sprouts			½ c	2.3	28
cabbage, red			½ c	1.4	15
cabbage, white			½ c	1.4	15
carrots			½ c	2.3	24
cauliflower			½ c	1.1	14
corn, canned			½ c	2.9	87
kale leaves			½ c	1.4	22
parsnip			½ c	2.7	51
peas			½ c	3.6	57
potato (w/o skin)			1 med.	1.4	97
potato (w/skin)			1 med.	2.5	106
spinach			½ c	2.1	21
squash, summer			½ c	1.4	13
sweet potatoes			½ med.	1.7	80
turnip			½ c	1.6	17
zucchini			½ c	1.8	11
raw					
bean sprout, soy			½ c	1.5	13
celery, diced			½ c	1.1	10
cucumber			½ c	0.4	8
lettuce, sliced			1 c	0.9	7
mushrooms, sliced			½ c	0.9	10
onions, sliced			½ c	0.8	33
pepper, green, sliced			½ c	0.5	9

DIETARY FIBER AND CALORIES FOR COMMON FOODS (continued)

FOOD	FIBER (GM)/ 100 GM*	CALORIES/ 100 GM	SERVING SIZE	FIBER (GM)/ SERVING	CALORIES/ SERVING
tomato			1 med.	1.5	20
spinach			1 c	1.2	8
LEGUMES					
baked beans, tomato sauce			½ c	8.8	155
dried peas, cooked			½ c	4.7	115
kidney beans, cooked			½ c	7.3	110
lima beans, cooked/canned			½ c	4.5	64
lentils, cooked			½ c	3.7	97
navy beans, cooked			½ c	6.0	112
BREADS, PASTAS, AND FLOURS					
bagels			1 bagel	0.6	145
bran muffins			1 muffin	2.5	104
cracked wheat			1 sl	1.0	62
crisp bread, rye			2 crackers	2.0	50
crisp bread, wheat			2 crackers	1.8	50
French bread			1 sl	0.7	102
Italian bread			1 sl	0.3	83
mixed grain			1 sl	0.9	59
oatmeal			1 sl	0.5	63
pita bread (5")			1 piece	0.4	123
pumpernickel bread			1 sl	1.0	66
raisin bread			1 sl	0.6	67

DIETARY FIBER AND CALORIES FOR COMMON FOODS (continued)

FOOD	FIBER (GM)/100 GM*	CALORIES/100 GM	SERVING SIZE	FIBER (GM)/SERVING	CALORIES/SERVING
white bread			1 sl	0.4	78
whole wheat bread			1 sl	1.4	61
pasta and rice (cooked)					
macaroni			1 c	1.0	144
rice, brown			1 c	1.0	97
rice, polished			½ c	0.2	82
spaghetti (regular)			1 c	1.1	155
spaghetti (whole wheat)			1 c	3.9	155
flours and grains					
bran, corn	62.2				
bran, oat	27.8				
bran, wheat	41.2				
rolled oats	5.7				
rye flour (72%)	4.5	350			
rye flour (100%)	12.8	335			
wheat flour:					
whole meal	8.9	318			
brown	7.3	327			
white	2.9	333			
NUTS					
almonds	7.2	627	10 nuts	1.1	79
peanuts	8.1	568	10 nuts	1.4	105
filberts	6.0	634	10 nuts	0.8	90

Over a period of months, such a removal of calories from the system could result in the steady loss of pounds.

Some researchers, however, have cautioned that the body may adjust to a high-fiber diet so that energy losses cease. If this is the case, the energy-loss mechanism may be only temporary and result in the reduction of a limited amount of body weight.

Finally, some fiber may alter the insulin responses in the body, which have been associated with obesity. Among other things, some studies have suggested that insulin levels may be reduced as fiber lowers certain insulin-controlling hormone levels in the stomach and intestines.

The exact ways that fiber works to fight obesity aren't always clear, but the final result is: There's a direct correlation between weight loss and the amount of fiber you consume, especially fiber containing guar gums (including oats, oat bran products, dried beans, and other legumes, such as peas and lentils).

THE 1,200-CALORIE CHALLENGE

So far, the information we've been considering may seem rather theoretical. You may find yourself thinking, "Okay, this high-fiber approach to weight loss has worked in scientific studies. But will it work for *me?*"

The answer is, emphatically, *yes!* To give you a brief introduction as to how well a high-fiber diet can work, try an experiment on yourself. This self-test, which I call the "1,200-calorie challenge," involves a personal evaluation for two days of how the quantity of food in a high-fiber diet compares with that in a low-fiber, high-fat diet.

The basic idea is to eat a low-fiber, high-fat diet one day, then a high-fiber, low-fat diet the next. (Caution: If you're already on a low-fat diet for health reasons, you should check with your physician to be sure that trying a high-fat regimen is acceptable.) Take notes periodically each day to record when and if you become hungry and the extent to which the meals satisfy you.

I've included sample meals for each of the two "challenge" days, one with high-fiber dishes and the other with low-fiber, higher-fat items. Each day provides for 1,200 calories, which is a comfortable amount for most people.

You can see just from looking over the foods listed for each day that the quantity is considerably higher on the high-fiber menu than on the low-fiber menu. The reason, as I've already said, is that it takes about twice as many carbohydrates to equal the calories in fat. Because high-fiber ingredients tend to be found primarily in carbohydrate-based dishes, you'll naturally find a greater quantity of food on the high-fiber day than on the low-fiber day.

Most likely, you'll feel less hungry after consuming the high-fiber diet because even though the calories are the same, your stomach will be filled up more easily. Also, you can eat more times during the day and thus satisfy your cravings when they strike without worrying about over-shooting your allotted number of calories.

THE LOW-FIBER DAY

Note: The following menu is *not* recommended, both because it contains too little fiber and because it is inherently unbalanced nutritionally. This one-day "challenge" is presented only to give the reader an idea of how unfavorably (and unfillingly) a low-calorie, low-fiber menu compares with a low-calorie, high-fiber menu.

BREAKFAST:
It's assumed that at each meal the dieter drinks water, black coffee, or some other liquid with no or minimal calories.

Eggs fried in butter (230 calories)	2 medium
Broiled bacon (90 calories)	1 slice
White toast (70 calories)	1 slice

LUNCH:

Tuna, white, water-packed (120 calories)	3 ounces
White bread (140 calories)	2 slices
Mayonnaise (100 calories)	1 tablespoon

SUPPER:

Hamburger patty (245 calories)	3 ounces
Hamburger bun (120 calories)	one, 3½-inch diameter
Raw tomato (20 calories)	½ medium
Tomato catsup (15 calories)	1 tablespoon
Graham crackers (55 calories)	2 squares

TOTAL FIBER FOR THE DAY: About 3 grams

THE HIGH-FIBER DAY

Note: This menu *is* recommended for those who want to lose weight. In fact, it's one of the days included in this book's weight-loss program—in Week 3, Day 3, on page 138.

BREAKFAST:
Low-calorie whole wheat French toast	2 slices
Low-calorie syrup	2 tablespoons
Skim milk	1 cup
Kiwi/strawberry fruit cup	1 cup

LUNCH:
Roast beef sandwich:
Roast beef	2 ounces
Sautéed onion/peppers	½ cup
French roll	1 each
Steak sauce	1 teaspoon
Mango	½ small
Skim milk	1 cup

SUPPER:
Tricolor Pasta Primavera with Chicken (see recipe on page 161)	1 serving
Lettuce salad	1 cup
Low-calorie dressing	2 tablespoons

SNACK *(in afternoon, before bed, or split between these two times):*
Green grapes	15 small

TOTAL FIBER FOR THE DAY: 19 grams

Now that you've had a taste of what it's like to go on a high-fiber weight-loss diet, you may be ready to embark on your own fiber-based weight-loss program. To this end, I've provided you with two weeks of sample menus at 1,200 calories a day to get you off on the right foot. These menus are included as a separate column in the menus section in Chapter 9. (You'll want to read Chapter 8 first to help you understand the basic strategy underlying the design of all the menus.)

As you try the weight-loss menus, keep these ideas in mind:

• The menus allow for approximately 1,200 calories a day. This amount of food is enough to ensure that you'll take in sufficient vitamins and minerals, yet the calories are low enough to enable you to lose at least two pounds a week.

• Always eat high-fiber foods first. This means focusing on vegetables, bran muffins, or other high-fiber items before you even consider eating anything else. Toward the end of a meal you may turn to higher-fat dishes—if you find you still have room in your stomach!

• For snacks, eat *only* high-fiber foods. This means bran products, raw vegetables, fresh fruits, or the like, *not* cookies or other sweets.

• Feel free to substitute equal calorie amounts of other high-fiber foods in these menus. You already have a chart showing fiber and calorie content of various foods. I know eventually you'll want to diverge from my suggestions and devise your own personal meal plan using this information.

The major benefit of a high-fiber diet has been discussed already—namely, a defense against high cholesterol, cancer, constipation, diverticulitis, and obesity. But the promise of fiber doesn't stop here, as will become evident in the following chapter.

6

A Potpourri of Present Benefits— And Future Promises

We've already explored many of the major benefits of a high-fiber eating plan, including the use of this food to prevent cholesterol problems and atherosclerosis, cancer, diverticulitis, constipation, and obesity.

But there's more. In this chapter, I'll provide you with the latest research and thinking on how fiber can help you overcome

- diabetes,
- gallbladder disease, and
- duodenal ulcers.

I'll also review how a high-fiber diet can be an extremely helpful tool in responding to the special concerns of athletes, children, and pregnant women. Finally, I'll discuss current research on the use of a high-fiber diet to combat such health problems as kidney disease.

THE DIABETES BENEFIT

Diabetes mellitus, the most common form of diabetes, is a condition caused by the inability of the body to burn off sugars that have been taken in through the diet. When you eat foods high in carbohydrates, the liver converts the sugars in these foods to glucose, another form of sugar used for energy.

The levels of glucose in the body are controlled by the hormone insulin, which is produced by the pancreas. Insulin allows the glucose, which is circulating in the bloodstream, to be utilized by the cells of the body.

If there isn't enough insulin or if the insulin isn't working properly, the glucose may go out of control (a condition known as hyperglycemia, or excess blood sugar). Diabetic symptoms include feelings of weakness, blurred vision, frequent urination, unusual loss of weight, and an almost insatiable thirst. In the most serious cases, the diabetes or excess glucose may damage organs, particularly the kidneys, and contribute to strokes and heart disease.

Diabetes is generally divided into two categories: insulin dependent and non–insulin dependent. The insulin-dependent type means that insulin must be introduced from outside the body to control the glucose; the non-insulin-dependent type may be controlled by other means. Another way of categorizing this disease is to identify it as juvenile, which is always insulin dependent, or adult onset, which may or may not be insulin dependent.

Fiber can provide a natural treatment for diabetes in a few ways. First, obesity is a major risk factor in much adult-onset diabetes. The more tissue the body has in the form of fat, the more insulin it needs to control the circulating glucose. In a number of cases, because the pancreas can't produce sufficient insulin to meet the needs of the fat cells in obese people, diabetes mellitus strikes. Consequently, there is a need to provide insulin from the outside, as in the form of insulin injections.

Conversely, leaner bodies have less fat and thus less need of insulin. Overweight adults, then, who are at risk can reduce their excess poundage through a high-fiber, lower-calorie diet.

Second, fiber inhibits or slows down the release of sugars contained in the foods we eat. Certain of the soluble fibers, such as pectin (in apples) and the guar gums (found in oatmeal, oat bran, dried beans, or other legumes), can perform this function.

Finally, a major danger confronting diabetics is the development of atherosclerosis, or the buildup of fatty plaque in blood vessels through the process popularly known as "hardening of the arteries." Atherosclerosis is promoted through a diet high in cholesterol and saturated fats. Yet a high-fiber diet will automatically provide relatively more complex carbohydrates and fewer fats.

Doctors used to prescribe a low-carbohydrate, high-fat diet for diabetics because they wanted to keep the intake of sugars by the body as low as possible. But more recent studies have prompted nutrition experts to emphasize a diet low in fats (to prevent atherosclerosis) and higher in complex carbohydrates, such as vegetables, fruits, and foods high in soluble fibers.

Why does a high-carbohydrate diet work so well for diabetics? Complex carbohydrates release their sugars more slowly than do simple carbohydrates, like candy or refined sugar. As a result, there tends to be less of a "rush" of sugars into the body. Also, high-carbohydrate diets are associated with lower, better-controlled concentrations of insulin in the blood.

Caution: If you have diabetic tendencies, you must not embark on any diet without first consulting with your physician. Choosing the wrong kind of diet for your particular needs could be dangerous.

The outlook is extremely bright, then, for diabetics or diabetic-prone individuals who embark on The Fiber Prescription. At present, studies show that adults with insulin-dependent (or Type 1) diabetes can lower their insulin requirements by an average of 40 percent if they eat a diet high in carbohydrates and fiber.

The promise of a high-fiber, high-carbohydrate diet is even more dramatic for adults with non-insulin-dependent (or Type 2) diabetes. They can expect to lower their insulin needs by up to 100 percent. Furthermore, in 90 percent of the cases, Type 2 diabetics can actually discontinue insulin from outside sources. (See James W. Anderson, "Dietary Fiber in Nutrition Management of Diabetes," *Dietary Fiber: Basic and Clinical Aspects.* New York: Plenum Press, 1986, p. 355.)

THE GALLBLADDER BENEFIT

I mentioned the link between cholesterol and the gallbladder in Chapter 2. But more needs to be said about how a high-fiber diet can help protect against that prevalent scourge, gallstones.

Gallstones—lumps of calcium, bile pigment, and/or cholesterol that form in the gallbladder—are one of the most common ailments in the United States and Europe. Up to 60 percent of women and 30 percent of men develop gallstones during their lifetimes. Yet this problem can often be prevented with fiber.

The effectiveness of a high-fiber diet in preventing gallstones has been established through a number of studies, such as a 1984 report in the *Japanese Journal of Medicine*. In that investigation, researchers determined that in patients with gallstones, the fat intake was 22 percent higher and the crude fiber intake was 18 percent lower than in a group without gallstones. They concluded that increases in gallstones were related to increases in the intake of dietary fat and decreases in fiber consumption.

How does a high-fiber diet fight gallbladder disease?

In a number of studies, increasing the amount of wheat bran (containing insoluble fiber) in the diet has been linked to a decrease in cholesterol saturation in human bile. Some researchers feel that the wheat bran helps deplete the bile's pool of deoxycholic acid, a substance that, in excessive quantities, has been associated with a high incidence of gallstones.

Another possible explanation relates to an argument I've already made in favor of soluble fibers, such as oat bran. As you know, these fibers help to bind the cholesterol in food and thus prevent it from being absorbed into the bloodstream through the intestinal tract.

Just as this action lowers the cholesterol in the blood and can prevent hardening of the arteries, it may also prevent cholesterol from collecting in the gallbladder. With less cholesterol available in the gallbladder, there would be less likelihood for gallstones to develop.

A third possible explanation focuses on fat. As you know, the more fiber you eat in your diet, the less animal fats you tend to consume. By lowering the fats you take in, you lower the total circulating lipids, including the cholesterol, in your blood. In this way—as with the binding action of fiber—there is less cholesterol available to be excreted through your bile, and thus less chance of your having gallstones.

It's no wonder, then, that doctors typically prescribe a low-fat, high-fiber diet for those with gallbladder problems.

THE DUODENAL ULCER BENEFIT

Several studies have demonstrated that a high-fiber diet may help prevent ulcers of the duodenum (the first part of the small intestine, which connects to the stomach).

For example, in 1982 Dr. Andreas Rydning of Lovisenberg Hospital in Oslo and several colleagues investigated patients with recently healed duodenal ulcers. They put one group on a high-fiber diet, including high-fiber breads, porridge, vegetables, and fruit. A second group of patients stayed on a low-fiber diet.

The results: During the six-month follow-up, only 45 percent of the patients on the high-fiber regimen had a recurrence of their ulcers, in comparison with 80 percent of those on the low-fiber diet.

In another study, reported in 1984 in *American Surgery*, researchers found that 5 grams of guar gum, which can be found in such foods as oatmeal, reduced the acidity level of gastric juices within a one- to two-hour period. The scientists concluded that a diet high in guar gums should be helpful to duodenal ulcer patients.

One report has cautioned that patients with an impeded outlet from the stomach (pyloric stenosis) may experience severe retention of food in the stomach with a guar gum diet.

There may also be limits on how much a high-fiber diet

can help heal duodenal ulcers that are active. So far, the only studies showing the benefits of this diet have dealt with preventing the condition.

THE FIBER PROMISE FOR ATHLETES, CHILDREN, AND PREGNANT WOMEN

There are some special fiber considerations that concern three groups we haven't discussed in detail—athletes, including amateurs of all ages who participate in regular vigorous exercise; children; and pregnant women.

Athletes

If you want to maintain a high energy level, especially during strenuous exercise, a high-carbohydrate diet is important. The reason is that your body stores energy in the form of glycogen in the liver and the muscles. As exercise or other outside activities place demands on you, the glycogen is released in response.

After you've used all the stores of glycogen, your body will switch to fat to provide the energy—and burning body fat, while it contributes to a loss of weight, is much less efficient than burning glycogen. The longer you can stay on glycogen, which may be likened to "high octane" bodily fuel, the better performance you can expect.

As we have seen already, high-carbohydrate foods tend to be high in fiber. Yet it's essential for athletes and other very active people to choose foods that have *usable* complex carbohydrates and that aren't simply high in fiber bulk.

In other words, if I stuffed athletes with such foods as celery and lettuce, they would have to eat huge quantities of these foods to get the calories they need. There is just too much indigestible fiber in some carbohydrates to provide enough energy to support vigorous, extended physical activity.

On the other hand, if I fed athletes pasta, such as spaghetti, their bodies would be able to break down this food and use it for energy. The reason: There is less indigestible fiber bulk in pasta than in many other complex carbohydrate foods, such as celery.

If you are an extremely active person and you find that you're running out of steam during a sports event or another strenuous time of the day, you probably just need more calories. The goal should be to choose such foods as pastas and add higher-calorie vegetables or fruits, like oranges, for a snack.

If you choose pasta as a snack, be careful about eating the usual high-fat foods, like cheese, that may accompany it. Remember, The Fiber Prescription emphasizes *fiber*, not fat.

Finally, a note on carbohydrate loading: This practice, which involves eating piles of pasta or similar foods high in complex carbohydrates before a race or athletic event, was popular a few years ago. But more recent training techniques emphasize eating high-carbohydrate meals regularly, not only before special events. This way, the body is ready to perform at a peak level during practice or ordinary daily activities, as well as during important competitions.

Children

An infant, whether breast-fed or bottle-fed, is literally on a zero-fiber diet. By the time the child reaches age 2, however, fiber will have become a significant part of his food program. Then, by age 4 or 5, he'll be on the regular family eating plan. That may create problems if Mom and Dad have become major fiber enthusiasts.

A word of advice: *Go slow!*

There are several reasons for caution. First of all, the gastrointestinal tract of a child is immature, so he's more likely to experience the discomfort of excess gas if he is on a high-fiber regimen.

Even more important, a diet that is very high in fiber may deprive a child of the nutrients he needs for full growth and development. Too much indigestible food may become a substitute for other essential nutrients. Furthermore, the fiber may bind minerals like zinc, calcium, and iron, which are necessary for proper growth.

A classic story of zinc deficiency emerged during a study in Egypt of children who were dwarfs or who experienced infantile sexual development. It turned out that both boys and girls in this group had a diet low in zinc. In addition, they had been eating the fiber phytate, common in some Middle Eastern diets. Phytate, which can be found in various cereals, whole meal products, and soybeans, binds zinc. Therefore, the little zinc the children were getting was being tied up by the fiber and prevented from entering their bodies. Their severe lack of development was the result.

Although zinc deficiency is much less of a problem in the United States, it does occur. Several studies in Colorado and other locations have established zinc deficiencies through tests on zinc in the hair and blood of children.

Fiber, especially insoluble fiber, may also bind calcium, which is essential for the development of strong bones. Children should take in at least 1,000 milligrams of calcium daily, but few get that amount. If they are on a high-fiber diet, what they do get may be washed out of their systems in bowel movements through the fiber-binding process.

The third problem with children and fiber concerns iron. Fiber may bind iron taken in through the diet and send it out of the body before it can enter the bloodstream. The result may be an iron deficiency with varying symptoms, anemia being the last stage. Other symptoms include a deterioration in work performance, a shortening of attention span, and a reduction in physical capabilities.

You can expect a child with even mild iron deficiency to experience a lessening of school performance. There will be an increasing inability to focus on a problem and stay focused on it.

Administering iron orally, through tablets, can produce a marked change in alertness and performance within a week or less. But the best approach to keeping iron up to adequate levels is to watch the child's diet and be sure that excess fiber or iron-poor foods aren't depleting the iron stores.

Iron deficiency is the most common nutritional problem among children, largely because as their blood supply increases with growth, their demands for iron steadily increase. It's a basic rule among pediatric nutritionists that the faster you grow, the greater your requirement for iron will be. Infancy, then, is the most important time for increasing iron, and adolescence is probably the second most important.

How much fiber can a child safely consume? Certainly, every child must take in an adequate amount of fiber to ensure easy and regular bowel movements and to condition the palate for increasing amounts of fiber later in life.

But again, I would urge you to *go slow*. Don't automatically put your child on the same high-fiber regimen you may be following.

I've recommended that adults shoot for 20 to 30 grams of fiber a day, but that's entirely too much for a young child. The best rule of thumb for adults is to consume a minimum of about 7 to 8 grams of fiber per 1,000 calories. That means that a man on a 3,000-calorie diet should be taking in at least 21 to 24 grams of fiber daily. Furthermore, most men at this calorie level could benefit from twice that much fiber a day.

But it's different with children. I recommend that children eat about 6 grams of fiber per 1,000 calories. Since some young children consume only 1,000 calories a day, their fiber limit is 5 to 6 grams—quite a difference from the 20- to 30-gram minimum I'm suggesting for adults.

If you embark on The Fiber Prescription, you'll have to make adjustments to accommodate your children. Just keep track of the amount of fiber they are consuming by checking the values in the charts in this book or on the labels of boxes and cans of food.

Then do some simple calculations: Find out the average number of calories they take in each day, divide by 1,000, and multiply by 6. That will give you the maximum number of grams of fiber your children should be eating. When growth has been completed after adolescence, children can start a regular high-fiber diet.

Example: Assume your children consume an average of 1,500 calories a day. Divide that figure by 1,000 to get 1.5. Then, multiply by 6 (grams of fiber) to get 9 grams of fiber, the maximum amount of fiber they should take in daily.

Pregnant Women

I've already discussed in Chapter 4 how pregnant women may experience constipation during pregnancy and how they can overcome this problem with a high-fiber diet.

A benefit of a high-fiber diet during pregnancy is control of cholesterol, which tends to rise after conception. The process of keeping cholesterol at acceptable levels for pregnant women is the same as that for anyone, as discussed in Chapter 2.

Caution: Because some rise in cholesterol levels in the mother-to-be is normal and may be important for the growth of the fetus, it's important not to go overboard in lowering cholesterol. In general, if the woman has had a cholesterol problem before pregnancy and has been following a high-fiber diet, it's acceptable to control the level of cholesterol through a reasonable high-fiber diet during pregnancy. Obviously, any dietary manipulations should be tried only under the supervision of a qualified physician.

Another benefit of a high-fiber diet during pregnancy is weight control. Women naturally gain weight while they are pregnant, but there is also a tendency in some women to gain too much—and to have tremendous difficulty getting rid of the excess pounds after they give birth. A high-fiber diet may be useful to such women as a way to satisfy their increased appetite without fostering obesity.

As with the cholesterol issue, a pregnant woman should *not* embark on a special weight-reduction or weight-control diet during pregnancy without close medical supervision.

CURRENT RESEARCH

The benefits of a high-fiber diet are many, and we can expect further benefits to be uncovered through research. Some thought is already being devoted to how fiber can be used to combat kidney disease, for instance. This area is currently the focus of considerable controversy. Data in animal research suggest that high-protein diets may be damaging to kidneys over a long period. Since any high-fiber regimen will tend to be a low-protein diet, depending on the fibers that are chosen for consumption, it is thought that a high-fiber diet should be incorporated in any treatment of kidney disease.

Other studies are being done to define the benefits and operations of specific types of fibers. At present, we are still searching for good, comprehensive definitions of fiber and a more precise understanding of how it works in the body.

In another decade or so we should have more news about how full-fiber menus can influence stomach cancer, cardiovascular disease, health problems of the elderly, and a host of other concerns. In the meantime, we have plenty of evidence to motivate us to stay on the high-fiber nutritional track.

7

Can Fiber Ever Be Dangerous?

If every member of industrialized Western societies embarked on a personal high-fiber nutritional strategy, many of the major diseases we face, such as heart problems and cancer, would decline. But as the old saying goes, there can always be too much of a good thing—and fiber is no exception.

There are indeed some potential disadvantages—and maybe even dangers—in a fiber diet that is excessive in some ingredients or that lacks proper nutritional balance. In general, I divide the possible drawbacks of fiber into two types: those that merely produce discomfort and those that are toxic, or poisonous, in some way to the body.

DODGING THE POSSIBLE DISCOMFORTS OF FIBER

Those who embark too rapidly on a high-fiber diet often develop gas pains, flatulence, and a sense of being bloated, but these problems usually decrease significantly or disappear within a few days. In a few people, the physical responses can be worse and may include nausea, diarrhea, and even vomiting.

Unfortunately, the negative responses can be sufficiently unpleasant to cause many people to go off a high-fiber regimen immediately. Yet if they were only patient and waited a few days—or at most, a week or so—their gastrointestinal tracts would adjust and the problems would go away.

A major goal I always emphasize to individuals who are just beginning on a high-fiber eating plan is to do all they can *at the outset* to minimize the unpleasant side effects of fiber. To this end, a simple but extremely important strategy for those who want to pursue this eating program— and continue to reap its many benefits—is to move slowly and be willing to backtrack. If you find you are experiencing some gas or stomach pains, just cut back on the amount of fiber you're eating.

The amount of fiber to cut from the menus is a highly individual decision, by the way. Human nutritional needs and physical side effects to a high-fiber diet vary greatly. So it's necessary to experiment with your food plan and decide for yourself: "Should I reduce the amount of bran in my cereal bowl?" Or "Should I eat one less muffin a day?"

Just be assured of this: If you have the patience to allow your body to adjust to this new food program, in almost every case the discomfort will disappear.

THE REAL DANGERS POSED BY THE WRONG APPROACH TO FIBER

In the discussion of fiber and children in the previous chapter, I mentioned several potential dangers that may be posed by a high-fiber diet. These included the binding of zinc, calcium, and iron and the failure of these nutrients to be absorbed in the body.

A similar kind of challenge may confront adults who are on a high-fiber program. As we'll see, though, a balanced fiber diet, which includes sufficient nutrients, can eliminate the possibility of any danger for most people.

Zinc

A 1984 study reported in *Human Nutrition* investigated the effect of wheat bran on zinc absorption in adults over a seven-day period. Volunteers who were fed 20 grams of wheat bran plus a zinc sulfate solution daily experienced a significant reduction in their absorption of zinc. The researchers concluded that the consumption of wheat bran at these levels, under these circumstances, could eventually induce a state of zinc deficiency.

Several other investigations have reached similar results. So what should we conclude from these studies?

The key to good health and to avoiding zinc deficiencies—as well as other types of nutritional deficiencies—while on a high-fiber diet seems to incorporate two basic principles: *balance* and *consistency*.

97

Specifically, a varied fiber diet helps prevent deficiencies that may result from the body's response to an overabundance of one type of fiber. When eaten to excess, for instance, some components of fiber, such as phytate, may bind zinc and cause inadequate amounts of this mineral to enter the body. (Phytate is a salt of phytic acid, which is formed from phytin, another salt that can be found in many seeds and tubers. Foods such as wheat cereals, whole meal products, and soybeans contain phytate.)

When too little zinc is being processed by the body, unusual fatigue or lethargy may result. But when integrated into a balanced nutritional program, the "dangerous" fiber products that have been binding zinc or other minerals or vitamins often lose their power to harm.

Staying on a well-designed high-fiber diet for weeks, months, or years gives the body time to adjust and to absorb nutrients that may have been prevented from absorption at the outset of the diet. For example, studies of vegetarians, who eat relatively high-fiber diets, have uncovered no problem with zinc deficiencies, most likely because experienced vegetarians tend to consume all sorts of fibers. Also, they have given their bodies plenty of time to adjust to a high-fiber regimen.

A case in point: In a 1981 study reported in the *American Journal of Clinical Nutrition,* fifty-six vegetarian women, whose average age was 53, were found to have adequate levels of zinc in their bodies. On the other hand, nonvegetarians in another 1981 study lost significant amounts of zinc while on a high-fiber vegetarian diet for twenty-two days.

You'll recall from the previous chapter that phytate has been implicated in binding zinc. The Egyptian children in the study discussed ate relatively high amounts of grain products and took in too little zinc and other minerals.

Fortunately, phytate isn't found in great quantities in our diet, but some breakfast cereals, such as those high in wheat bran, do contain this substance. Consequently, although a sensible meal plan should include cereals high in bran fiber, there should also be a focus on foods with little or no phytate, such as most vegetables and fruits. In addition, it's important to take in plenty of foods like meats, which contain iron and zinc.

Remember, the ultimate goal is *balance:* Too much beef *or* fiber will backfire nutritionally. The precise amount you need of each is an individual matter that you and your physician must determine. In general, however, my recommendation of 20 to 30 grams a day of fiber, along with less than 30 percent of calories from fats, should be adequate for most people.

Iron

The study cited above in the *American Journal of Clinical Nutrition* also investigated the effect of a high-fiber vegetarian diet on levels of iron. The results were similar: A high-fiber vegetarian diet followed over several years had no negative implications for the absorption of iron into the body.

The addition of whole wheat bread to one's diet has been found to inhibit the absorption of iron into the body. But when iron-rich foods (e.g., meat or fish) are added to the meal, the loss of iron can be prevented.

In general, when high amounts of fiber are added to a balanced diet, there doesn't seem to be much of an effect on iron absorption into the body. Problems seem to arise only when high amounts of bran are consumed *without* counterbalancing nutrients from high-protein beans, vegetables, meats, poultry, or fish.

Calcium

There has been ongoing concern that a high-fiber diet may deplete the body of calcium, especially among children, pregnant women, lactating women, and the elderly, who have special needs for this mineral. The recommended daily allowance (RDA) for calcium is 800 milligrams, but 1,000 milligrams a day is preferable. For children, pregnant women, lactating women, and the elderly (who are at higher risk of osteoporosis), 1,500 milligrams a day of calcium is the best goal.

The concern about calcium depletion has prompted several studies that have shed some light on the subject. For example, in a 1983 report in the *American Journal of Clinical Nutrition*, twelve men ate three separate diets for four weeks each. One diet involved 5 grams of fiber a day with spinach; another included 27 grams of fiber a day with spinach; a third involved 27 grams of fiber a day with cauliflower (instead of spinach).

The results: At the end of the fourth week, the average balance of calcium was significantly lower after the high-fiber diet with spinach. The researchers concluded that the combination of a high-fiber diet, combined with the oxalic acid in spinach, had an adverse effect on the body's calcium.

A big problem in getting enough calcium on a high-fiber diet is often not the binding effect of fiber, but rather the substitution of fiber for other nutrients. As you have learned, the substitutionary role of fiber can work to your advantage as you rid your diet of high-fat foods. But it's important not to eliminate high-calcium foods, such as skim milk or nonfat yogurt.

The concerns expressed in this chapter about the binding effect on minerals of different types of bran have been included for one main reason: It won't do just to follow advice that says, "Eat plenty of fiber!"

Instead, you need a comprehensive plan, a program that offers plenty of the *right kind* of fiber *plus* other necessary nutrients. A major goal of The Fiber Prescription is to maximize the benefits of fiber, which include the prevention of various diseases and conditions that are currently devastating the health of many in our society. At the same time, this diet should ensure that you absorb plenty of zinc, iron, and calcium, as well as other important vitamins and minerals.

8

Your Personal Strategy for Putting Fiber First

The time has arrived to put into practice all the facts you've been learning about fiber. In this chapter, I'll provide you with a step-by-step plan to make this important food the foundation of your personal nutrition. To show you what's possible in your own kitchen, let's take a look at how one woman managed to sift through all the scientific gobbledegook about fiber and actually launch a high-fiber eating program.

HOW HELEN DEVELOPED A FIBER PRESCRIPTION FOR HER FAMILY

Helen was confused.

She had a history of colon cancer in her family. Her husband, Hal, was overweight, had a cholesterol problem, and had been diagnosed as being at high risk for heart disease. And Helen herself suffered periodic bouts with constipation. She knew that a large part of the answer to these health concerns might be a high-fiber diet, but she was puzzled about how to formulate an effective meal program for her family.

Helen had studied various books and articles on fiber, listened to lectures on the subject, even consulted with a registered dietitian. But she still didn't understand how to design a meal plan to maximize the potential health benefits that she knew a high-fiber diet could offer.

Some of the questions that bothered her:

"We want to benefit from all the advantages that are available from the different types of fiber. How can I reach an appropriate balance of soluble and insoluble fiber?"

"How can we avoid the danger of toxic effects from too much fiber?"

"What's the best balance between high-fiber sources like cereals, vegetables, legumes, and fruits?"

There was also an immediate reason that Helen was concerned. She had started to increase her family's fiber intake and found that both she and her husband were experiencing the typical initial reactions of excessive gas, loose bowel movements, and occasional stomach pains. Hal finally declared that he couldn't continue on this track: "Let's find a way to eat fiber without all the side effects, or let's forget it!" he said.

What Helen really needed was a plan. Finally, with the help of a physician friend who understood nutrition and was sympathetic to her plight, she settled on an approach that worked like this:

• Helen assembled everything she knew about the foods that contain various kinds of fiber. Then she selected a representative sampling of items she and Hal liked that contained relatively high levels of soluble and insoluble fiber.

The foods high in soluble fiber included oat bran muffins, baked beans, and lentil soup. Also important were apples, which contain pectin, a soluble fiber. The foods high in insoluble fiber included wheat bran cereals, broccoli, brussels sprouts, and cauliflower.

• Using these and other favorite foods, Helen planned high-fiber menus that contained roughly equal amounts of insoluble and soluble fiber. She designed them around the goal of 20 to 30 grams of fiber a day. (In a few pages, you'll see how to do this yourself by referring to certain charts I've included in this chapter.) As she had throughout her long experience as the family cook, Helen made sure that each day's meals were well balanced, with all the basic vitamins and minerals her family needed.

• Contrary to the approach she had first used, Helen introduced the high-fiber foods *gradually*. She and Hal discovered that they could minimize the side effects of a high-fiber regimen by eating only 15 grams of fiber a day for the first week or so. (Like most Americans, they had been eating about 11 grams of fiber a day under their old, lower-fiber approach.)

After about three weeks, Helen and Hal discovered that their systems had adjusted to the extra amounts of fiber. At that point, they were able to take in a full 20 to 30 grams of fiber a day without discomfort.

The results have been gratifying. Now, about a year later, Helen has no more problems with constipation. As for Hal, he's lost about ten pounds, and his cholesterol has dropped from 260 mg/dl to 210 mg/dl. By most measures,

both are at much lower risk for colon cancer and a variety of other health problems.

What can we learn from the experience of Helen and Hal? I would suggest the following two-step plan, which should launch you successfully on The Fiber Prescription.

STEP 1: REVIEW YOUR KNOWLEDGE OF FIBER

You already have an extensive knowledge of fiber from your previous reading in this book. This first step is merely intended to encourage you to review much of what you already know and to provide you with more practical information that will help you in your selection of high-fiber foods.

How Much Fiber?

To begin with, remember the general guideline I suggested in the very first chapter of this book: Your target should be to take in 20 to 30 grams of fiber a day.

It's probably wise not to consume more than 35 grams of fiber a day unless you're an experienced vegetarian who knows how to ensure a proper balance of important nutrients. Adding huge amounts of fiber (in excess of 35 grams) indiscriminately may crowd other important foods out of your diet and may produce too many unwanted side effects, such as gas and diarrhea.

Soluble vs. Insoluble

Next, it's necessary to distinguish between soluble and insoluble fiber—that is, fiber that is soluble or not soluble in water.

You'll recall that soluble fiber and insoluble fiber perform somewhat different jobs in your body, though there is some overlap in function. For example, soluble fiber has been associated with binding and lowering cholesterol in the blood. Insoluble fiber is linked strongly to decreasing the transit time of the stool in the colon, thus relieving constipation and lowering the risk of colon cancer. (Soluble fiber can also help improve bowel movements.)

Because both types of fiber perform important operations in the body and because there is some overlap in their benefits, I believe it's important to include both types of fiber in your diet. How much should you have of each? I would recommend trying roughly for a 50–50 split. That is, focus about half of your fiber intake on those foods known to contain high amounts of soluble fiber and half on foods with insoluble fiber.

How can you tell which foods contain soluble fiber and which contain insoluble fiber? Food labels, when they refer to fiber, usually don't distinguish between soluble and insoluble, and many high-fiber foods contain both soluble and insoluble fibers.

To help you out, here are some of the most common foods in each category:

Soluble-fiber foods include those with pectin, gums, and hemicellulose, such as oats, oat bran, oatmeal, apples, citrus fruits, strawberries, dried beans, barley, rye flour, potatoes, raw cabbage, and pasta. (These have been as-

sociated with lower cholesterol in the blood, as well as with softer bowel movements.)

Insoluble-fiber foods include those with cellulose, lignin, and hemicellulose, such as wheat bran, whole wheat products, cereals like All-Bran and Shredded Wheat, mature vegetables, barley, grain, whole wheat pasta, and rye flour. (These are linked to protection from colon cancer, diverticulitis, and constipation.)

For a more precise idea of the relative amounts of soluble and insoluble fiber in certain foods, see the accompanying charts.

Some pointers to understanding the charts: The gram amounts of fiber given for each food item represent the number of grams of fiber in every 100 grams (or 3.5 ounces) of the listed food.

The letters *NCP* stand for non-cellulose polysacharides, or fibers that lack cellulose fiber. Cellulose, you'll recall, is the sugar-based, insoluble fiber that constitutes a large part of the cell walls of plants. NCP fibers may be either soluble or insoluble.

You can get a general idea of the total soluble fiber in each food by referring to the "Soluble NCP" line and a general idea of the total insoluble fiber by adding the "Cellulose" and "Insoluble NCP" lines.

The "Total" line after each food item indicates the total grams of the three types of fiber combined in every 100 grams (3.5 ounces) of the listed food.

At this point, I'm just providing you with some tools for later use in meal planning. I would suggest that you look over these charts and be familiar with the foods and information contained in them. But don't try to memorize anything at this point or make any final decisions. That would be premature and might just cause confusion.

When we reach the point of actually talking about what

SOLUBLE AND INSOLUBLE FIBER CONTENT IN SELECTED FOODS

FOOD	TYPE OF FIBER	GRAMS OF FIBER
All-Bran	Cellulose	4.67
	Soluble NCP	3.94
	Insoluble NCP	15.22
	Total	23.83
Cooked potato	Cellulose	1.63
	Soluble NCP	2.64
	Insoluble NCP	0.57
	Total	4.84
Corn bran	Cellulose	16.70
	Soluble NCP	6.57
	Insoluble NCP	55.21
	Total	78.48
Cornflakes	Cellulose	0.24
	Soluble NCP	0.18
	Insoluble NCP	0.23
	Total	0.65
Haricot beans (dry)	Cellulose	4.20
	Soluble NCP	7.20
	Insoluble NCP	5.38
	Total	16.78
Iceberg lettuce	Cellulose	7.17
	Soluble NCP	9.35
	Insoluble NCP	2.72
	Total	19.24
Instant potato	Cellulose	1.61
	Soluble NCP	2.89
	Insoluble NCP	0.24
	Total	4.74
Oats	Cellulose	0.48
	Soluble NCP	4.86
	Insoluble NCP	2.25
	Total	7.59

SOLUBLE AND INSOLUBLE FIBER CONTENT IN SELECTED FOODS *(continued)*

FOOD	TYPE OF FIBER	GRAMS OF FIBER
Pearl barley	Cellulose	0.36
	Soluble NCP	4.77
	Insoluble NCP	2.66
	Total	7.79
Porridge oats	Cellulose	0.41
	Soluble NCP	4.51
	Insoluble NCP	2.15
	Total	7.07
Raisins	Cellulose	0.58
	Soluble NCP	1.12
	Insoluble NCP	0.19
	Total	1.89
Raw cabbage	Cellulose	9.86
	Soluble NCP	13.53
	Insoluble NCP	4.21
	Total	27.60
Raw potato	Cellulose	1.77
	Soluble NCP	2.76
	Insoluble NCP	0.61
	Total	5.14
Rice	Cellulose	0.26
	Soluble NCP	0.32
	Insoluble NCP	0.04
	Total	0.62
Rye bread	Cellulose	0.39
	Soluble NCP	1.76
	Insoluble NCP	1.00
	Total	3.15
Rye flour	Cellulose	1.49
	Soluble NCP	4.61
	Insoluble NCP	7.80
	Total	13.90

SOLUBLE AND INSOLUBLE FIBER CONTENT IN SELECTED FOODS *(continued)*

FOOD	TYPE OF FIBER	GRAMS OF FIBER
Soy isolate	Cellulose	—
	Soluble NCP	0.35
	Insoluble NCP	0.62
	Total	0.97
Wheat bran	Cellulose	5.89
	Soluble NCP	3.51
	Insoluble NCP	22.81
	Total	32.21
White flour	Cellulose	0.19
	Soluble NCP	1.96
	Insoluble NCP	1.05
	Total	3.20
White wheat flour	Cellulose	0.24
	Soluble NCP	0.94
	Insoluble NCP	0.65
	Total	1.83
Whole wheat bread	Cellulose	1.61
	Soluble NCP	2.67
	Insoluble NCP	5.63
	Total	9.91
Whole wheat flour	Cellulose	1.77
	Soluble NCP	1.83
	Insoluble NCP	6.19
	Total	9.79

SOURCE: Adapted from Hans N. Englyst and John H. Cummings, "Measurement of Dietary Fiber as Nonstarch Polysaccharides," in *Dietary Fiber: Basic and Clinical Aspects,* ed. by George V. Vahouny and David Kritchevsky. New York: Plenum Press, 1986.

FIBER CONTENT OF SOME CEREAL PRODUCTS

FOOD	TYPE OF FIBER (GRAMS)				TOTAL GRAMS
	CELLULOSE	SOLUBLE	INSOLUBLE		
White bread	0.13	1.91	0.59		2.63
White flour	0.16	1.58	0.86		2.60
White bread crust	0.14	1.81	0.61		2.56
White bread crumb	0.18	1.73	0.67		2.58
Brown bread	1.06	2.33	3.85		7.25
Brown flour	1.29	2.19	4.53		8.01
Brown bread crust	1.03	2.90	3.49		7.42
Brown bread crumb	1.23	2.69	3.78		7.70
Whole meal bread	1.52	2.57	5.48		9.58
Whole meal flour	1.57	2.55	6.03		10.15
Whole meal crust	1.35	3.07	5.00		9.42
Whole meal crumb	1.65	2.86	5.49		10.00
Wheat bran, Arjuna	8.17	4.25	28.60		41.06
Wheat bran, Allinson's Broad Bran	7.98	3.22	30.37		41.57
All-Bran (Kellogg's)	4.38	3.94	15.36		23.68
Weetabix	1.59	3.28	5.54		10.41
Shredded Wheat	1.70	2.33	6.70		10.73
Cornflakes	0.26	0.18	0.24		0.68
Rice Krispies	0.40	0.20	0.29		0.89
Oatmeal, medium ground	0.40	3.93	2.96		7.29

FIBER CONTENT OF SOME CEREAL PRODUCTS *(continued)*

FOOD	TYPE OF FIBER (GRAMS)			TOTAL GRAMS
	CELLULOSE	SOLUBLE	INSOLUBLE	
Scott's Porage Oats	0.28	3.98	2.96	7.22
Rye grain	1.52	4.47	7.24	13.23
Rye flour	1.40	4.61	7.68	13.69
Barley grain	1.44	3.89	6.50	11.83
White rice, round grain	0.16	0.16	0.35	0.67
Brown rice	0.70	0.14	1.18	2.02
White rice, long grain	0.21	0.13	0.24	0.58
Sago	0.35	0.26	—	0.61
Digestive Wheatmeal biscuits	0.33	1.38	1.26	2.97
Rich Tea biscuits	0.14	1.58	0.50	2.22
Semolina	0.31	1.22	1.06	2.59
Macaroni	0.28	1.59	1.11	2.98
Spaghetti	0.20	1.85	0.97	3.02
Spaghetti, whole wheat	1.78	2.42	5.75	9.95
Tapioca	0.08	0.13	0.23	0.44
Arrowroot	0.01	0.03	0.02	0.06

SOURCE: Englyst, H.N., Anderson, V., and Cummings, J.H., "Starch and non-starch polysaccharides in some cereal foods," *Journal of Scientific Agriculture,* vol. 34 (1983) pp. 1434–1440.

foods you'll include in your meal program, things will become simpler—and the charts will become much clearer. You'll then be able to rely heavily on the menus and recipes that are included in this book and use them as a model to select certain favorite foods, like a specific brand of bran cereal, apples, oranges, baked beans, or broccoli, and make those the staples of your diet.

STEP 2: DEVELOP YOUR OWN PERSONAL STRATEGIES FOR SELECTING AND PREPARING HIGH-FIBER FOODS

You now have an idea about how a number of common foods fit into the soluble- and insoluble-fiber categories. Also, you know that half of your fiber intake should consist of soluble fiber and half of insoluble fiber. Finally, you realize that it's important to keep your total consumption of fiber each day in the range of 20 to 30 grams.

The time has come to start putting high-fiber foods on your table. To this end, I'd recommend that you use the following suggestions to design your own personal strategies for buying, preparing, and eating high-fiber foods.

Strategy #1: Employ the Simplest Approach to Selecting and Buying High-Fiber Foods.

You should decide the types of high-fiber foods you prefer after considering what has been said in this text, including the menus and recipes in the following chapters. Then make a list of your favorites and post it in the kitchen. Be sure to stock up regularly on those high-fiber foods so that you'll always have some on hand when you're preparing a meal or looking for a snack.

Here are some guidelines to keep in mind:

• Because dietary fiber is found in foods that come from plants, you can forget about the supermarket sections with dairy products, meats, and oils. Instead, check out the aisles with cereals, breads, grains, vegetables, and fruits.

• Be aware that serving sizes listed on labels may vary. In evaluating fiber content, check the packages to be sure that the serving size listed is what you expect to eat. Many whole-grain cereals contain about 2 grams of dietary fiber per serving, while bran cereals are higher. Some high-fiber cereals contain 12 to 14 grams per serving.

• The serving size for bread is usually one slice. Whole wheat breads provide about 1 to 2 grams of fiber a slice. But manufacturers of some low-calorie breads add extra fiber, so these products may contain between 2 and 3 grams of fiber per serving.

• Noodles, spaghetti, and brown rice typically supply about 1 gram of fiber per ½ cup (cooked) serving. Prepared grains, barley, and cracked wheat supply about 3 grams per ½ cup (cooked) serving.

• A typical serving size for fruits is ½ cup canned or juice, 1 cup fresh. One cup of fresh fruit will usually supply about 2 grams of fiber. Higher-fiber fruits include apples, blackberries, currants, mangoes, pears, raspberries, and rhubarb, which provide about 4 grams per serving. Juices contain much less fiber than an equivalent amount of fresh fruit.

• The usual serving size for vegetables is 1 cup raw, ½ cup cooked. These foods usually provide about 2 grams of fiber per serving. Vegetables that are quite high in fiber include broccoli, brussels sprouts, okra, and turnips, which supply about 4 grams per serving.

• As for beans and legumes, a typical serving is ½ cup cooked. Like bran, beans can supply a large amount of dietary fiber, especially the soluble kind. Each serving supplies 5 to 6 grams of fiber. Kidney and butter beans supply about 7 grams per serving.

A further word about food labels: Unfortunately, when labels do mention fiber (and, of course, with items like fresh fruits and vegetables there are no labels), they rarely distinguish between soluble and insoluble fiber. Consequently, you should try to go into the supermarket with a prior understanding of what foods are high in the different types of fiber.

Strategy #2: Establish and Follow a Plan for the Times that You Eat Fiber.

Although it's necessary to set a target for consuming 20 to 30 grams of fiber each day, it's also important to decide *when* you'll eat it. As a rule, you should take in part of your daily fiber as part of each meal. This way, the soluble fiber in your diet can act directly and immediately to bind the cholesterol in your gastrointestinal tract. Also, the insoluble fiber you eat will be better able to hurry the other foods through your system.

High-fiber items can also be quite helpful as snacks between meals. Because the transit time to get food through your system involves hours, extra fiber both before and after a meal can help provide your stomach and intestines with a "fiber bath" and streamline the action of the gastrointestinal tract.

For example, suppose you eat lunch at 1:00 P.M., have a bran muffin at 3:00 P.M., and eat your dinner at 6:00 P.M. In this case, the fiber in the muffin would hasten the movement of the lunch food and would also pave the way for a faster processing of the evening meal.

Remember, too, that many foods contain the kinds of fiber you need. You might begin the day with oatmeal, wheat bran, or a combination of oat bran (or oatmeal) and wheat bran. In addition, you might add an oat bran or wheat bran muffin. This way, you'd start out with both soluble and insoluble fiber.

Then, you could have a helping of vegetables or fruit for lunch, perhaps along with another bran muffin. In the middle of the afternoon, you might eat an apple or an orange to take in some soluble fiber. Finally, at dinner you should eat plenty of vegetables and perhaps some fruit for dessert.

By spreading your fiber intake throughout the day and by dividing the types of fiber more or less equally between soluble and insoluble, you'll be on your way to enjoying the full benefits of a full-fiber diet.

A note on concentrated fibers: For most people, I don't recommend the consumption of concentrated fibers, such as pure oat bran or liquid extracts. It's always best to take in nutrients through regular foods because they taste better and can be merged more naturally into the average meal. The concentrated fibers may seem dry or unappetizing, and in fact, when taken alone, they often taste like medicine! A major component of my philosophy of high-fiber eating is to make fiber an integral part of eating, not an extraneous, sprinkled-on addition to other dishes.

Sometimes, though, concentrated fibers may be helpful either because a person simply can't take in enough food during the day to get sufficient fiber or because a physician recommends the supplement. In such situations, it's extremely important to monitor the exact amount of fiber so as not to take in too much.

Strategy #3: Feel Free to Adjust Your Diet to Accommodate Special Nutritional Needs.

A high-fiber diet is a very flexible eating program that can be fine-tuned to meet a variety of individual needs. Two questions that I'm frequently asked by those interested in embarking on a fiber-centered diet are these:

What do I do if I'm a vegetarian?

The answer: Keep on eating just as you're eating! By definition, a vegetarian diet is a high-fiber diet.

Of course, there may be a few minor adjustments you'd like to make, such as incorporating more soluble fiber like oat bran into your diet. Most likely, though, you're already experiencing the benefits of a high-fiber diet, such as lower blood pressure and cholesterol levels, easy and regular bowel movements, successful weight control, and a lower risk of colon cancer and diverticulitis.

As you've undoubtedly noticed, most of the foods I've mentioned as high-fiber foods are those normally included in a vegetarian regimen, such as fresh fruits, vegetables, and whole-grain products. If you'll turn to the next chapter and glance briefly at the menus and recipes there, you'll find them literally packed with vegetarian fare. In fact, the meals on Day 7 of Week 2 (in both the 2,000- and 1,200-calorie diets) are vegetarian.

What do I do if I'm lactose intolerant?

Those who are lactose intolerant have an inability to digest the milk sugar lactose in dairy products because of deficiencies in the enzyme lactase. In other words, a lactase deficiency leads to lactose intolerance. The symptoms may include excessive gas, diarrhea, cramps, and other uncomfortable gastrointestinal reactions.

You'll note that the model menus in the next chapter

include skim milk, yogurt, and other dairy products. The main reason for this is to ensure that those on the diets get at least the minimum recommended daily allowance (RDA) of 800 milligrams of calcium.

The dairy products have been spread out through the day to ease the impact on those who are lactose intolerant. Even though many people have this problem, it's present in varying degrees. That is, a few people react violently to *any* milk. But most have an internal threshold that allows them to take in a certain amount of dairy products without triggering the symptoms. They can drink *some* milk or eat *some* yogurt without ill effects.

If you find that you still have reactions to the minimal amounts of milk sugar, you'll probably have to switch to a calcium supplement. One of the most common is calcium carbonate. Some people with a very low level of stomach acid, however, find that this supplement doesn't dissolve properly and thus fails to enter their system in adequate amounts. Another popular supplement is calcium citrate, which several studies have shown to be more available biochemically to those with low amounts of stomach acid.

In any event, before you start taking any supplement, you should consult your physician.

Strategy #4: Get Started Immediately in Preparing and Eating High-Fiber Foods.

Beneficial, long-term change occurs in our lives only when we put down a book like this and begin to take action. The time is now! The next two chapters will provide you with some model menus, recipes, and other guidelines to help you launch your exciting, high-fiber nutritional adventure.

9

Full-Fiber Menus and Recipes

By now you've identified some of the high-fiber foods you think you'd like to eat and started thinking seriously about a basic eating strategy. The next step is to begin the actual process of preparing and serving meals.

To help you design a practical meal plan, I've included three weeks of 2,000-calorie menus and three weeks of 1,200-calorie weight-loss menus. Obviously, you'll want to vary these menus to fit your own individual style of eating. But the basic approach, with balanced nutrients and high-fiber dishes, should be maintained.

The 2,000-calorie menus have been designed for weight *maintenance* for the average person. Some women may find they have to eat less to maintain their present weights, while some active or large men may find they have to take in more calories to stay at the same weight.

The 1,200-calorie menus are a weight-*loss* program that should allow the average man or woman to lose about two pounds per week. You should check with your physician before going on any weight-loss regimen, but this calorie

119

level is adequate to allow most people to proceed without direct medical supervision.

In using these menus or others that you may formulate yourself, it's important to keep in mind several principles:

• When you prepare a high-fiber dish, including such mundane items as oatmeal, *do not pour off excess water* that accumulates during preparation. Remember: Much fiber is soluble; that is, it dissolves in water. If you eliminate the water, you'll also be eliminating a great deal of soluble fiber.

• Be sure to drink eight to nine 8-ounce glasses of fluids each day. Water and other noncaffeinated, noncarbonated drinks are the best sources. Milk may also be all right, so long as no one in the family has a lactose intolerance. Coffee, tea, and sodas may help replenish lost fluids, but the caffeine and other substances they contain may make them undesirable sources of liquids for many people.

• The most common foods that contain the highest amounts of fiber tend to be bran cereals (but check labels to be sure how much fiber you get per serving!). These cereals do not have to be limited to breakfast. Many people who are trying to lose weight or who are having trouble getting their fiber intake up to the desired level eat cereals as a snack or as a major part of another meal.

• Soups can be a significant source of fiber, but be sure to analyze the fiber content before you make any soup a staple of your diet. For example, bean soups, such as lentil, can be excellent sources of fiber, while broth or cream soups are not.

We're ready to move on to the actual menus and recipes, which are described in the following two sections.

ABOUT THE MENUS

Calorie and fat values for recipes were taken from *Food Values of Portions Commonly Used* by Jean Pennington (New York: Harper & Row, 1989) and package labels.

Dietary fiber values for recipes and menus were taken from *Plant Fiber in Foods* by James Anderson, M.D., H.C.F. (Nutrition Research Foundation, Inc., 1990), Pennington's *Food Values*, and package labels.

Calorie and fat levels of daily menus were estimated using the American Diabetes Association and the American Dietetic Association's Exchange Lists for Meal Planning, 1986. All menus follow the American Heart Association's guidelines limiting dietary fat to approximately 30 percent of daily calories.

Abbreviations used in the menus and recipes are as follows:

> ctn—carton
> g—gram
> cal—calorie
> lg—large
> med—medium
> oz—ounce
> sml—small
> svng—serving
> tbsp—tablespoon
> tsp—teaspoon

Full-Fiber Menus

Week One, Day One

BREAKFAST	2,000 CAL	1,200 CAL
Cracked wheat cereal with	1 cup	½ cup
Raisins	2 tbsp	———
Skim milk	1 cup	1 cup
Whole wheat toast	1 slice	1 slice
Margarine	1 tsp	1 tsp
Orange juice	½ cup	½ cup

LUNCH		
*Butter bean casserole	2 svng	1 svng
Saltine crackers	6	6
Watermelon chunks	1¼ cups	1¼ cups
Skim milk	1 cup	1 cup

DINNER		
Grilled chicken breast	4 ounces	3 ounces
*Lemon vegetables	2 svng	1 svng
Baked potato	1 small	———
French roll	1 each	1 each
Margarine	1 tsp	———
*Rhubarb cake	1 svng	———
Low-calorie gelatin	———	½ cup

SNACK		
Peanut butter	1 tbsp	1 tbsp
Apple, quartered	1 med	1 med

TOTAL FIBER CONTENT (g)	33	18

*Recipe provided

Week One, Day Two

	2,000 CAL	1,200 CAL
BREAKFAST		
*Oat bran zucchini muffin	2	1
Plain low-fat yogurt	1 cup	1 cup
Citrus fruit cup	1 cup	½ cup
LUNCH		
Ham sandwich:		
Sliced ham	3 ounces	2 ounces
Lettuce and tomato slices	3	3
Whole wheat bread	2 slices	———
Low-calorie whole wheat bread	———	2 slices
*Kidney bean salad	1 svng	1 svng
Banana	½ sml	½ sml
DINNER		
Spaghetti	2 cups	1 cup
Meatballs (1 oz ea)	2	1
Parmesan cheese	2 tbsp	2 tbsp
Lettuce and tomato salad with	2 cups	1 cup
Dressing or	1 tbsp	———
Low-calorie dressing	———	1 tbsp
Skim milk	1 cup	1 cup
SNACK		
Mango	1 sml	½ sml
Wheat crackers	5 each	———
TOTAL FIBER CONTENT (g)	23	17

*Recipe provided

Week One, Day Three

BREAKFAST	2,000 CAL	1,200 CAL
Shredded wheat	1 cup	———
Puffed wheat	———	1 cup
Skim milk	1 cup	1 cup
Whole wheat toast	2 slices	1 slice
Margarine	1 tsp	1 tsp
Jelly (any flavor)	1 tbsp	———

LUNCH		
*Hot bean and chicken salad with	1 svng	1 svng
Mixed greens	1 cup	1 cup
Bagel	2 halves	———
Margarine	1 tsp	———
Fruit cocktail	½ cup	———
Low-calorie gelatin	———	1 cup

DINNER		
Roast beef	5 ounces	3 ounces
*Winter vegetable sauté	2 svng	1 svng
Mashed potato	1 cup	½ cup
Margarine	1 tsp	1 tsp
*Winter fruit compote	1 svng	1 svng

SNACK		
Plain low-fat yogurt	1 cup	1 cup

TOTAL FIBER CONTENT (g)	29	16

*Recipe provided

Week One, Day Four

BREAKFAST	2,000 CAL	1,200 CAL
*Bake 'em as you need 'em muffins	2	1
Margarine	2 tsp	———
Low-fat buttermilk	1 cup	1 cup
Applesauce	———	½ cup

LUNCH		
Roast beef sandwich:		
Roast beef	3 ounces	3 ounces
French roll	2	1
Mayonnaise	1 tsp	———
Steak sauce	———	2 tbsp
Pear	———	1 sml
*Minted pears	1 svng	———
Skim milk	1 cup	1 cup

DINNER		
Grilled chicken leg	2	1
*Curried peas and carrots with	2 svng	1 svng
Brown rice	⅔ cup	⅓ cup
*Oriental salad	1 svng	1 svng
Gingersnaps	3	1

SNACK		
Pretzels	1½ ounces	¾ ounce
Cantaloupe cubes	1 cup	1 cup

TOTAL FIBER CONTENT (g)	26	15

*Recipe provided

Week One, Day Five

BREAKFAST	2,000 CAL	1,200 CAL
Shredded wheat with	1 cup	————
Raisins	2 tbsp	————
Puffed wheat	————	1 cup
Skim milk	1 cup	1 cup
Grapefruit	½	½

LUNCH		
*Greek beans	2 svng	1 svng
Reduced-fat cheese on	1 ounce	1 ounce
French bread	2 slices	1 slice
Margarine	2 tsp	————
Lettuce salad and	2 cups	1 cup
Dressing or	2 tbsp	————
Low-calorie dressing	————	2 tbsp
Plums	2 med	2 med

DINNER		
Broiled fish	5 ounces	3 ounces
*Stir-fried spinach with sesame seeds	1 svng	1 svng
*Bulgur pilaf	1 svng	1 svng
Vanilla wafers	6	————

SNACK		
Graham crackers	6	3
Skim milk	1 cup	1 cup

TOTAL FIBER CONTENT (g)	33	20

*Recipe provided

Week One, Day Six

BREAKFAST	2,000 CAL	1,200 CAL
*Oatmeal pancakes with	2	2
Syrup or	2 tbsp	——
Low-calorie syrup	——	2 tbsp
Margarine	2 tsp	1 tsp
Orange juice	½ cup	½ cup
Low-calorie fruit yogurt	1 ctn	1 ctn

LUNCH		
*Vegetarian vegetable soup	2 svng	1 svng
Ham sandwich:		
Ham slices	2 ounces	——
Mayonnaise	1 tsp	——
Tomato and lettuce slices	3	——
Whole wheat bread	2 slices	——
Whole wheat melba toast	——	5 slices
Sherbert (any flavor)	¼ cup	——
Low-calorie gelatin	——	½ cup

DINNER		
Broiled pork chop	3 ounces	3 ounces
*Broccoli, orange, and red pepper salad	1 svng	1 svng
Baked potato	1 large	1 sml
Margarine	2 tsp	1 tsp

SNACK		
Cottage cheese	½ cup	½ cup
Sliced peaches	2 halves	2 halves

TOTAL FIBER CONTENT (g)	24	15

*Recipe provided

Week One, Day Seven

BREAKFAST	2,000 CAL	1,200 CAL
Oatmeal with	½ cup	½ cup
Raisins	2 tbsp	2 tbsp
Skim milk	1 cup	1 cup

LUNCH		
*Garbanzo bean salad over	2 svng	1 svng
Lettuce	2 cups	1 cup
Celery and carrot sticks	1 cup	1 cup
French roll	2	1
Cantaloupe cubes	1 cup	1 cup
Skim milk	1 cup	1 cup

DINNER		
Broiled lean hamburger with	5 ounces	3 ounces
Sautéed mushrooms on	1 cup	½ cup
Hamburger roll	2 halves	———
*Pineapple parsnips	2 svng	1 svng
Fresh cherries	12	12

SNACK		
Breadsticks	2	2
Reduced-fat cheese cubes	2 ounces	1 ounce
Grapes	15 sml	———

TOTAL FIBER CONTENT (g)	25	16

*Recipe provided

Week Two, Day One

BREAKFAST	2,000 CAL	1,200 CAL
Creamy hot oat bran cereal with	¾ cup	¾ cup
Sliced banana	1 sml	½ sml
Toast	1 slice	———
Margarine	1 tsp	———
Skim milk	1 cup	1 cup

LUNCH		
*Vegetarian vegetable soup	2 svng	1 svng
Saltine crackers	6	———
Tuna salad on	¾ cup	½ cup
Whole wheat bread	2 slices	1 slice

DINNER		
*Pepper steak stir-fry over	1 serving	1 serving
Brown rice	1 cup	⅔ cup
Fresh peaches sprinkled with powdered ginger	2 halves	2 halves

SNACK		
Low-calorie fruit yogurt	1 ctn	1 ctn

TOTAL FIBER CONTENT (g)	28	18

*Recipe provided

Week Two, Day Two

	2,000 CAL	1,200 CAL
BREAKFAST		
Branflakes with	½ cup	½ cup
Raisins	2 tbsp	———
Bagel with	1 whole	———
Cream cheese	1 tbsp	———
Fresh orange	1 whole	1 whole
Skim milk	1 cup	1 cup
LUNCH		
Lentil soup	1 cup	1 cup
French bread	1 slice	———
Mozzarella cheese slices	2 ounces	1 ounce
Mixed green salad with	2 cups	2 cups
Dressing or	1 tbsp	———
Low-calorie dressing	———	2 tbsp
DINNER		
*High-fiber meatloaf	1 svng	¾ svng
Baked potato	1 sml	1 sml
Corn	½ cup	———
Kiwi	1	1
Skim milk	1 cup	1 cup
Margarine	1 tsp	1 tsp
Carrots	———	½ cup
*Oatmeal cookie	1	———
SNACK		
Whole strawberries	1¼ cup	1¼ cup
TOTAL FIBER CONTENT (g)	29	24

*Recipe provided

Week Two, Day Three

BREAKFAST	2,000 CAL	1,200 CAL
*Oatmeal pancakes with	3	2
Syrup or	1 tbsp	———
Low-calorie syrup	———	2 tbsp
Margarine	2 tsp	———
Blueberries	2 cups	1 cup
Skim milk	———	1 cup

LUNCH		
*Chicken salad with	1½ svng	1 svng
Whole wheat pita pocket	1	1
Carrot/celery sticks	1 cup	1 cup
Apple	1 small	———
Skim milk	1 cup	½ cup
Vanilla wafers	6	———

DINNER		
*Quick chili with	1 svng	1 svng
String cheese	2 sticks	1 stick
Mixed green salad and	2 cups	2 cups
Dressing or	1 tbsp	———
Low-calorie dressing	———	2 tbsp
French roll	1	———
Melon balls	1 cup	1 cup

SNACK		
Graham crackers	3	3
Skim milk	1 cup	½ cup

TOTAL FIBER CONTENT (g)	22	15

*Recipe provided

Week Two, Day Four

BREAKFAST	2,000 CAL	1,200 CAL
Whole wheat French toast with	2 slices	———
Syrup	2 tbsp	———
Light whole wheat French toast with	———	2 slices
Low-calorie syrup	———	2 tbsp
Low-fat plain yogurt with	1 cup	1 cup
Sliced strawberries	¾ cup	¾ cup
LUNCH		
*Italian-style bean soup	2 svng	1 svng
*Spinach salad with	1 svng	1 svng
Dressing or	2 tbsp	———
Low-fat dressing	———	2 tbsp
Skim milk	———	1 cup
French roll	1	———
DINNER		
*Sweet and sour meatballs over	1 svng	1 svng
Brown rice	⅔ cup	⅓ cup
*Dilled green beans	1 svng	1 svng
*Peach crisp	1 svng	———
SNACK		
Mozzarella cheese	1 ounce	———
Whole wheat crackers	5	———
Low-calorie gelatin	———	1 cup
TOTAL FIBER CONTENT (g)	25	18

*Recipe provided

Week Two, Day Five

BREAKFAST	2,000 CAL	1,200 CAL
*Oat bran zucchini muffin	1	1
Grapefruit	½ whole	½ whole
Skim milk	1 cup	1 cup

LUNCH		
Turkey/mozzarella sandwich:		
Turkey	2 ounces	1 ounce
Mozzarella cheese	1 ounce	1 ounce
Mild pepper rings†	free**	free
Tomato slices	4	4
Mayonnaise or	2 tsp	———
Low-calorie mayonnaise	———	½ tbsp
Whole wheat bread or	2 slices	———
Light whole wheat bread	———	2 slices
Tomato juice	½ cup	½ cup
Nectarine	1 med	———
Skim milk	1 cup	1 cup

DINNER		
*Bran-fried fish fillets	1 svng	¾ svng
*Four-bean salad	1 svng	1 svng
*Orange sweet potatoes	1 svng	½ svng
Angel food cake (1½-in slice)	1	———
with canned cherries	½ cup	———

SNACK		
Pretzels	1½ ounces	———
Nectarine	———	1

TOTAL FIBER CONTENT (g)	24	19

*Recipe provided   **free—eat as many as you wish.
  †These are a pickled prepared product that add flavor but insignificant calories.

Week Two, Day Six

	2,000 CAL	1,200 CAL
BREAKFAST		
All-Bran cereal	⅓ cup	⅓ cup
Whole wheat toast	2 slices	————
Orange	1 med	1 med
Skim milk	1 cup	1 cup
Margarine	2 tsp	————
LUNCH		
*Minestrone soup	1 svng	1 svng
Meatloaf sandwich:		
*High-fiber meatloaf	¾ svng	½ svng
Whole wheat bread or	2 slices	————
Light whole wheat bread	————	2 slices
Catsup/steak sauce	2 tsp	2 tsp
Skim milk	1 cup	————
Fresh plums	2 sml	2 sml
DINNER		
*Bami goreng	1 svng	¾ svng
Fried banana	1 sml	½ sml
Rice cake	2 each	————
SNACK		
Low-fat frozen yogurt	⅔ cup	————
Low-calorie fruit yogurt	————	1 ctn
TOTAL FIBER CONTENT (g)	32	29

*Recipe provided

Week Two, Day Seven

BREAKFAST	2,000 CAL	1,200 CAL
Egg sandwich:		
Poached egg	2	1
Canadian bacon	2 ounces	½ ounce
English muffin	1 whole	1 half
Orange juice	½ cup	½ cup

LUNCH		
*Italian-style bean soup	1 svng	1 svng
Seven-grain bread or	1 slice	———
Light whole wheat bread	———	1 slice
Mixed green salad and	2 cups	2 cups
Dressing or	1 tbsp	———
Low-calorie dressing	———	2 tbsp
Skim milk	1 cup	1 cup
Apple	1 med	———

DINNER		
*Pepper steak stir-fry over	1 svng	1 svng
Brown rice	1 cup	⅓ cup
Gingersnaps	3	———
Mandarin oranges	¾ cup	¾ cup

SNACK		
Shredded wheat cereal	1 cup	½ cup
Skim milk	1 cup	1 cup
Blackberries	¾ cup	¾ cup

TOTAL FIBER CONTENT (g)	26	20

*Recipe provided

Week Three, Day One

BREAKFAST	2,000 CAL	1,200 CAL
*Apricot-bran muffin	1	1
Citrus fruit cup	1 cup	½ cup
Skim milk or low-fat plain yogurt	1 cup	1 cup

LUNCH		
*Quick chili-stuffed potatoes with	1 svng	1 svng
Reduced-fat cheddar cheese	1 ounce	½ ounce
Tossed salad and	2 cups	2 cups
Dressing or	1 tbsp	———
Low-calorie dressing	———	2 tbsp
French roll	1	———
Margarine	1 tsp	———
Pear with cinnamon	½ cup	½ cup

DINNER		
*Lemon chicken	1 svng	1 svng
*Wild rice and barley pilaf	2 svng	1 svng
Steamed broccoli	1 cup	½ cup
Margarine	1 tsp	———
Ice milk	1 cup	———
Raspberries	1 cup	1 cup

SNACK		
Shredded wheat fruit squares	½ cup	———
Skim milk	1 cup	1 cup
Low-calorie gelatin	———	1 cup

TOTAL FIBER CONTENT (g)	34	25

*Recipe provided

Week Three, Day Two

BREAKFAST	2,000 CAL	1,200 CAL
Low-fat plain yogurt	1 cup	½ cup
Cracked wheat cereal with	1 cup	½ cup
Cherries	½ cup	½ cup
Whole wheat toast	1 slice	———
Margarine	1 tsp	———
Berry preserves	1 tsp	———

LUNCH		
Pizza:		
Whole wheat bread or	4 slices	———
Light whole wheat bread	———	2 slices
Spaghetti sauce	4 tbsp	2 tbsp
Mozzarella cheese	3 ounces	2 ounces
Toppings:	1 cup	½ cup
Mushroom, tomato,		
olive, green pepper, etc.		
Skim milk	1 cup	1 cup

DINNER		
*Ham and potatoes florentine	1 svng	1 svng
Cooked carrots	½ cup	½ cup
Whole wheat bread	1 slice	———
Margarine	2 tsp	1 tsp
Cantaloupe cubes	1 cup	1 cup

SNACK		
Apple	1 med	1 med
Peanut butter	1 tbsp	———
Wheat crackers	———	5

TOTAL FIBER CONTENT (g)	31	23

*Recipe provided

Week Three, Day Three

BREAKFAST	2,000 CAL	1,200 CAL
Whole wheat French toast	2 slices	———
with syrup	2 tbsp	———
Light whole wheat French	———	2 slices
toast with		
Low-calorie syrup	———	2 tbsp
Skim milk	1 cup	1 cup
Kiwi/strawberry fruit cup	1 cup	1 cup

LUNCH		
Roast beef sandwich:		
Roast beef	2 ounces	2 ounces
Sautéed onion/peppers	½ cup	½ cup
Mixed grain bread	2 slices	———
French roll	———	1
Steak sauce	1 tsp	1 tsp
*Garbanzo bean salad	1 svng	———
Mango	½ sml	½ sml
Skim milk	1 cup	1 cup

DINNER		
*Tricolor pasta primavera	1 svng	1 svng
with chicken		
Lettuce and	1 cup	1 cup
Dressing or	1 tbsp	———
Low-calorie dressing	———	2 tbsp
Low-fat frozen yogurt	⅔ cup	———

SNACK		
Green grapes	15 sml	15 sml
Breadsticks	2	———

TOTAL FIBER CONTENT (g)	21	19

*Recipe provided

Week Three, Day Four

BREAKFAST	2,000 CAL	1,200 CAL
Branflakes with	½ cup	½ cup
Sliced nectarine	1	1
Raisin bagel with	1 whole	——
Cream cheese	1 tbsp	——
Skim milk	1 cup	1 cup

LUNCH		
*Italian-style bean soup	1 svng	——
Ham sandwich:		
Boiled ham	3 ounces	2 ounces
Tomato slices	3	3
Whole wheat bread or	2 slices	——
French roll	——	1
Mayonnaise or	1 tbsp	——
Low-calorie mayonnaise	——	1 tbsp
*Broccoli, orange, and red	2 svng	1 svng
pepper salad		
Skim milk	1 cup	1 cup
Fruit cocktail	½ cup	½ cup

DINNER		
*Halibut with vegetables in	1 svng	1 svng
lime marinade		
*Brown rice pilaf	2 svng	2 svng
Gelatin or	½ cup	——
Low-calorie gelatin	——	½ cup
Sliced bananas	1 sml	½ sml

SNACK		
Whole-grain cereal squares	½ cup	½ cup

TOTAL FIBER CONTENT (g)	28	21

*Recipe provided

Week Three, Day Five

BREAKFAST	2,000 CAL	1,200 CAL
Low-calorie fruit yogurt	1 ctn	1 ctn
English muffin or	1 whole	———
Light whole wheat toast	———	1 slice
Margarine	1 tsp	1 tsp
Berry preserves	1 tsp	1 tsp
LUNCH		
Broiled lean hamburger on	3 ounces	3 ounces
Whole wheat roll	1 whole	———
Catsup/steak sauce	2 tsp	2 tsp
Corn on the cob (6 in)	1	1
Margarine	1 tsp	———
*Winter vegetable sauté	1 svng	1 svng
Skim milk	1 cup	1 cup
Whole strawberries	1¼ cup	1¼ cup
DINNER		
*Confetti vegetable enchiladas	2 svng	1 svng
*Fast spanish rice	1 svng	1 svng
Sliced pineapple	⅔ cup	⅓ cup
SNACK		
Assorted sliced vegetables: Mushroom, carrot, broccoli, green pepper, etc.	1 cup	1 cup
Low-calorie ranch dressing as dip	———	2 tbsp
Ranch dressing as dip	1 tbsp	———
TOTAL FIBER CONTENT (g)	28	20

*Recipe provided

Week Three, Day Six

BREAKFAST	2,000 CAL	1,200 CAL
Oat bran cereal with	¾ cup	¾ cup
Brown sugar and	1 tsp	1 tsp
Raisins	2 tbsp	2 tbsp
Orange	1 med	1 med
Toast	1 slice	————
Margarine	1 tsp	————
Skim milk	1 cup	1 cup

LUNCH		
Baked beans over	1 cup	½ cup
*Polenta	¾ cup	¾ cup
Tossed salad and	2 cups	2 cups
Dressing or	1 tbsp	————
Low-calorie dressing	————	2 tbsp
Whole wheat crackers	5	————
Skim milk	1 cup	1 cup
Sherbert	¼ cup	————

DINNER		
Roast turkey	4 ounces	3 ounces
*Herbed barley	2 svng	1 svng
Peas	½ cup	½ cup
Cranberry sauce	2 tbsp	————
French roll	1	————
Margarine	1 tsp	————
Red grapes	15 sml	15 sml

SNACK		
Air-popped popcorn with	3 cups	1½ cups
Margarine	1 tsp	1 tsp

TOTAL FIBER CONTENT (g)	32	24

*Recipe provided

Week Three, Day Seven

BREAKFAST	2,000 CAL	1,200 CAL
Swiss cheese/mushroom omelet:		
Egg substitute	¾ cup	½ cup
Swiss cheese	1 ounce	1 ounce
Sliced mushrooms	½ cup	½ cup
Onion	¼ cup	¼ cup
Red/green pepper slices	½ cup	½ cup
Whole wheat toast	2 slices	———
Light whole wheat toast	———	2 slices
Margarine	2 tsp	———
Low-fat margarine	———	2 tsp
LUNCH		
*Confetti vegetable enchiladas	1 svng	———
with shredded lettuce	1 cup	———
*Vegetarian vegetable soup	———	1 svng
Mixed green salad and	———	2 cups
Low-calorie dressing	———	2 tbsp
Papaya	1 cup	1 cup
Vanilla wafers	6	———
Skim milk	1 cup	1 cup
DINNER		
*Marinated tomato and shrimp pasta	1 svng	1 svng
*Savory brussels sprouts	½ cup	½ cup
Skim milk	1 svng	1 svng
Red apple	1 med	1 med
SNACK		
Raisin bagel	1 whole	———
Cinnamon applesauce	1 cup	½ cup
TOTAL FIBER CONTENT (g)	26	20

*Recipe provided

Full-Fiber Recipes

COOKING WITH DRY BEANS

Beans are an excellent fiber source. While canned and frozen products are available (some of the former are specified in the recipes), you may wish to prepare your own beans. Of the several possible techniques, two are given here for soaking and cooking the beans. Plan to allow anywhere from 3 hours to 1 day to prepare your beans for serving. (Please note that some dry beans do not require these lengthy soaking/cooking times. For example, lentils, black-eyed peas, and split peas cook quickly without soaking.) Dry beans require a large amount of water for soaking and cooking. They will expand greatly: 1 cup of dry beans will swell to 2 to 3 cups cooked. Soaking 1 cup of dry beans will require about 6 to 7 cups of water.

Traditional Soaking Method

Put the beans in a large pot with a large amount of cold water. Cover and let the beans stand at room temperature for about 8 hours. You will need to refrigerate beans if you let them soak longer than this. The beans will swell to two to three times their original size. Drain and rinse the beans, then cook them.

Quick Soaking Method

Put the beans in a large pot with a large amount of cold water. Bring water to a boil and cook beans for 5 minutes.

145

Cover the pot, turn off the burner, and let the beans stand for 1 hour. Drain and rinse the beans, then cook them.

Cooking Method

1. Put the soaked beans in a large pot with water to cover, and cook for about ½ hour. Drain and rinse the beans.

2. Again put the soaked beans in water to cover. At this point, you can add seasonings and some oil for flavor (the oil also helps to prevent foaming). Cook beans until tender, from 1 to 2 hours, depending on the type of bean. (Note that soybeans are exceptions. They frequently take longer to soak and cook.) Do not add tomatoes, lemon juice, or vinegar until the beans are almost tender, as these will delay the softening process.

Italian-Style Bean Soup

½ cup shelled fresh peas
½ cup diced carrot
1 clove garlic, peeled and
finely chopped
1 tablespoon olive oil
One 14-ounce can
Italian-style tomatoes
Two 19-ounce cans cannellini
beans, undrained

2 cups chicken stock
½ cup fresh corn kernels
½ cup diced fresh green
beans
½ small head escarole,
washed and chopped
2 tablespoons flat-leaf parsley
½ cup freshly grated
Parmesan cheese

Cook the peas and diced carrot separately in boiling water until not quite tender. Drain and set aside. In a soup pot, sauté chopped garlic in olive oil until golden. Add tomatoes, one can of beans, including liquid, the chicken stock, peas, carrot, corn kernels, and green beans. Simmer over medium heat. Purée the second can of beans, with its liquid, in a blender, and add to the soup. Stir in the escarole. Bring soup to a boil, lower heat, and simmer for 10 minutes. Garnish each serving with chopped parsley and grated cheese.

Serves 10

Per serving: 118 cal, 4 g fat, 3 g fiber

Fast preparation tip: One 10-ounce package of frozen mixed Italian-style vegetables may be substituted for fresh vegetables.

Minestrone

Two 14½-ounce cans chicken
broth, or 3½ cups fresh
homemade chicken broth
One 15-ounce can kidney
beans, rinsed and drained
1 cup mixed fresh
vegetables, such as diced
carrots and green beans,
shelled peas, and corn
kernels
1½ pounds fresh spinach,
washed, quickly blanched,
drained very well, and
chopped
½ cup chopped onion

½ cup small pasta, such as
shells or bow ties
1 teaspoon dried basil
¼ teaspoon pepper
1 clove garlic, peeled and
pressed or minced
½ teaspoon olive oil
One 16-ounce can
Italian-style stewed
tomatoes
1 tablespoon balsamic
vinegar
1 teaspoon Worcestershire
sauce

Combine all ingredients in a soup pot and stir well to mix. Bring
to a boil, reduce heat, and simmer for 15 minutes.

Serves 4

Per serving: 256 cal, 3 g fat, 6 g fiber

Fast preparation tip: Substitute 1 cup frozen mixed vegetables
for fresh. Substitute one 10-ounce package frozen chopped
spinach for fresh.

Vegetarian Vegetable Soup

½ cup chopped onion
½ cup chopped celery
½ cup chopped peeled turnip
1 cup sliced peeled carrot
1 cup chopped cabbage
One 17-ounce can
  whole-kernel corn,
  undrained

1 cup diced peeled potato
1½ quarts water
Salt and pepper
One 16-ounce can stewed
  tomatoes
2 cups cut fresh green beans

Combine all ingredients except tomatoes and green beans in a soup pot. Cover and simmer gently for 20 minutes. Add tomatoes and green beans and continue to simmer for another 20 minutes.

Serves 6 to 8

Per serving: 105 cal, 1 g fat, 5 g fiber

Quick Chili

**One 15½-ounce can kidney
  beans**
½ pound lean ground beef
1 cup canned tomato purée
1 tablespoon minced onion

1½ tablespoons chili powder
½ teaspoon dried oregano
Freshly ground black pepper
**2 tablespoons chopped fresh
  cilantro**

Drain kidney beans, reserving ⅓ cup liquid. In a large skillet, brown ground beef lightly. Drain off fat. Add beans, tomato purée, onion, reserved liquid, chili powder, oregano, and black pepper, stirring to mix. Bring to a boil, lower heat, cover, and simmer for 10 minutes. Garnish with chopped cilantro.

Serves 4

Per serving (¾ cup): 252 cal, 8 g fat, 4 g fiber

Sweet and Sour Meatballs

1½ teaspoons honey mustard
**1 teaspoon finely chopped
  fresh tarragon, or ½
  teaspoon dried tarragon**
½ teaspoon cinnamon
**Salt and freshly ground
  black pepper to taste**

**1 pound lean ground beef, or
  1 pound ground turkey**
**1 cup whole berry cranberry
  sauce**
1 cup sauerkraut

In a bowl, blend mustard, tarragon, cinnamon, salt, and pepper. Add beef or turkey and mix gently but thoroughly. Form mixture into small balls.

Brown meatballs well in a lightly oiled skillet. Rinse sauerkraut; drain completely, pressing out as much liquid as possible. Add to skillet. Break up cranberry sauce and stir it in. Gently mix all ingredients, rolling meatballs around in the sauce, and simmer over low heat until bubbling. Serve over brown rice as a main dish, or alone as a hot appetizer.

Serves 4 to 6

Per serving (4 meatballs): 435 cal, 16 g fat, 0 g fiber

High-Fiber Meatloaf

1 pound lean ground beef
1 pound ground veal
1 cup oat bran
1 teaspoon chopped fresh thyme, or ½ teaspoon dried thyme

Freshly ground black pepper
2 egg whites
½ cup prepared barbecue sauce with onion bits, plus additional for coating

Preheat oven to 350°F.

Mix all ingredients gently but thoroughly. Pack in a 9¼ by 5¼ by 2¾-inch nonstick loaf pan. Coat top with about 2 more tablespoons barbecue sauce, if you wish. Bake for 45 minutes to 1 hour.

Serves 6, with leftovers for sandwiches

Per serving (4 ounces): 344 cal, 18 g fat, 2 g fiber

Pepper Steak Stir-Fry

2 tablespoons low-sodium
  soy sauce
1 tablespoon dry sherry
1½ teaspoons brown sugar
Approximately 2 tablespoons
  vegetable oil
3 large onions, peeled and
  cut in eighths
2 cloves garlic, peeled and
  minced

1 teaspoon minced fresh
  gingerroot
3 green or red bell peppers,
  cored, seeded, and cut into
  1-inch pieces
12 ounces flank or sirloin
  steak, sliced thin

In a cup, mix soy sauce, sherry, and brown sugar. Heat a large
skillet or wok, and in as little oil as possible stir-fry the onions,
garlic, and gingerroot until onions are golden and tender; remove
from skillet or wok and set aside. Add a bit more oil to the skillet
and stir-fry the peppers until they are tender-crisp. Remove peppers and add them to onion mixture. Over brisk heat, stir-fry the
sliced steak in two batches, until browned. Return the onion and
pepper mixture to the skillet and toss quickly. Add the soy sauce
mixture, stir to blend, and serve at once with brown rice.

(This dish may be thickened with 1 teaspoon cornstarch dis-
solved in 1 tablespoon cold water, stirred until smooth. Just
before serving, stir into the skillet over medium heat until liquids
thicken.)

Serves 4

Per serving: 246 cal, 16 g fat, 3 g fiber

Other good stir-fry combinations include:

Cubed boneless chicken breast
Diced onions
Sliced mushrooms
Cubed zucchini

      *   *   *

Sliced beef or chicken
Green cabbage, cut into ½-inch chunks

      *   *   *

Beef or chicken
Broccoli florets
Green onions (tops and bulbs)

      *   *   *

Strips of beef or chicken
Sliced fresh mushrooms, or shiitake mushrooms (soak in warm water for ½ hour, drain, remove stems, and slice)
Snow peas

Seasoning options include:

Minced garlic
Minced fresh gingerroot
Low-sodium soy sauce
Dry sherry
Hoisin sauce
Oriental oyster sauce
Black bean sauce or salted black beans, rinsed in a sieve and crushed
Oriental mustard
Sesame oil
Sesame paste, or tahini, or smooth peanut butter

Ham and Potatoes Florentine

2 teaspoons vegetable oil
1 cup chopped onion
1 cup chopped green pepper
2 cups peeled, sliced new
   potatoes, parboiled until
   nearly tender
One 14½-ounce can stewed
   tomatoes

1½ pounds fresh spinach,
   washed, cooked quickly,
   very well drained, and
   chopped
2 cups cubed ham
¼ cup freshly grated
   Parmesan cheese

Heat oil in a large nonstick skillet. Sauté onion and green pepper until soft. Add potatoes and tomatoes and simmer for a few minutes. Add spinach and ham and heat through. Sprinkle with grated cheese and serve immediately.

Serves 6

Per serving: 274 cal, 13 g fat, 3 g fiber

Fast preparation tip: Substitute one 10-ounce package frozen chopped spinach, thawed and well drained, for fresh. Substitute one 16-ounce can sliced potatoes, drained, for fresh.

Lemon Chicken

½ cup freshly squeezed
   lemon juice
⅓ cup soy sauce
½ cup white wine
1 clove garlic, peeled and
   minced or pressed

2 teaspoons crushed dried
   rosemary
⅓ cup minced onion
4 skinless, boneless chicken
   breast halves, about 4
   ounces each

Preheat oven to 350°F.

In a shallow baking dish, mix the lemon juice, soy sauce, wine, garlic, rosemary, and minced onion. Add the chicken breasts and enough water to cover them. Bake for 45 minutes.

Serves 4

Per serving: 158 cal, 3 g fat, 0 fiber

Hot Bean and Chicken Salad

1 medium carrot, peeled and shredded
½ small onion, peeled and chopped
1 stalk celery, sliced
¾ cup water
⅓ cup vinegar
1½ tablespoons sugar
1½ tablespoons cornstarch
1 beef bouillon cube, or 1 teaspoon beef bouillon granules
½ teaspoon celery seed
One 16-ounce can black beans, rinsed and drained
One 16-ounce can red kidney beans, rinsed and drained
½ cup diced cooked chicken

In a nonstick skillet coated with vegetable spray, stir-fry the carrot, onion, and celery for 2 minutes. Remove from heat. Combine water, vinegar, sugar, cornstarch, bouillon granules, and celery seed in a small bowl. Add this mixture to the skillet. Return to medium-high heat and cook, stirring, until bubbly. Add drained beans and chicken; simmer a few minutes until heated through.

Serves 4

Per serving: 277 cal, 3 g fat, 7 g fiber

Fast preparation tip: Substitute one 5- to 6-ounce can of chunked chicken, drained, for diced cooked chicken.

Bami Goreng
(Noodles Indonesian Style)

1 pound wheat linguine
3 large onions, peeled and
   coarsely chopped
2 cloves garlic, peeled and
   minced
2 tablespoons vegetable oil
1 small head cabbage, cored
   and coarsely chopped
   (about 4 cups, loosely
   packed)

3 cups shredded cooked
   chicken or lean ham
2 tablespoons Indonesian
   ketjap manis,* or
   low-sodium soy sauce
2 dried chile peppers
   (optional), seeded and torn
   into small pieces

Cook linguine according to package directions, drain thoroughly, and keep warm.

In a large skillet, sauté onions and garlic in oil until golden. Add cabbage and stir-fry until it is tender. Add chicken or ham and ketjap manis or soy sauce and toss just until heated through. Combine with linguine, stir until well mixed, and sprinkle with chile peppers if you like. Serve at once.

Serves 8

Per serving (with ketjap manis): 297 cal, 6 g fat, 3 g fiber

*Available at oriental food stores and many large supermarkets, or make from the following recipe:

Ketjap Manis

1 cup firmly packed brown
   sugar
1 cup water
¾ cup soy sauce

⅓ cup molasses
Pinch ground coriander
Black pepper to taste

Combine brown sugar and water in 1-quart saucepan and bring to a boil. Reduce heat to moderate and stir until sugar dissolves. Increase heat and boil for about 5 minutes, or until thickened slightly. Reduce heat to a simmer, stir in remaining ingredients, and simmer 3 minutes. Store in a glass jar in the refrigerator; it will stay fresh for 2 weeks.

Makes 1 pint

Per pint: 868 cal

Chicken Salad with Whole Wheat Pita Pockets

2 tablespoons reduced-calorie
   mayonnaise-type salad
   dressing
Dash garlic powder
2 teaspoons minced onion

½ teaspoon celery seed
1 cup cooked, diced chicken
   without skin
½ cup chopped celery

Mix salad dressing, garlic powder, onion, and celery seed in a bowl. Stir in chicken and celery and mix well. Serve in whole wheat pita pockets.

Serves 4

Per serving (without pita): 169 cal, 8 g fat, 0 g fiber

Halibut with Vegetables in Lime Marinade

1 pound thick-cut halibut
  steaks
½ cup freshly squeezed lime
  juice
1½ tablespoons olive oil
1 clove garlic, peeled and
  minced
1 teaspoon chopped fresh
  oregano leaves, or ½
  teaspoon dried oregano

2 teaspoons chopped fresh
  basil leaves, or ½ teaspoon
  dried basil
Water or dry white wine
½ cup broccoli florets
1 cup coarsely diced carrots
1 medium zucchini, diced in
  ½-inch cubes
1 cup whole cherry tomatoes
½ teaspoon grated lime rind

Cut fish into 1-inch cubes and place in a shallow glass or enamel dish. Mix lime juice, olive oil, garlic, and herbs and pour over fish. Add water or wine to barely cover the halibut cubes. Marinate 30 to 60 minutes in the refrigerator.

Steam or microwave broccoli, carrots, and zucchini briefly, until tender-crisp. Mix these and the cherry tomatoes with the fish and its marinade.

Microwave in a covered casserole dish on high for 4 minutes, or poach in the marinade in a covered skillet until fish flakes easily, about 8 minutes. Sprinkle with grated lime rind and serve hot.

Serves 4

Per serving: 173 cal, 7 g fat, 2 g fiber

Bran-Fried Fish Fillets

4 fish fillets of equal size
  (about 2 pounds), such as
  sole or walleye
Low-fat milk to cover
3 egg whites
1 cup oat bran
1 tablespoon snipped fresh
  dill, or 1½ teaspoons dried
  dill

1 teaspoon paprika
Salt (optional)
Freshly ground black pepper
3 tablespoons safflower oil
Lemon wedges
Chopped fresh parsley

Place fish fillets in a shallow glass or enameled dish and cover with milk. Refrigerate for 1 hour.

Beat egg whites in a shallow dish until frothy. Combine oat bran, dill, paprika, salt, and pepper on a large sheet of wax paper.

Drain fish and pat dry on paper towels. Dip fillets first into egg whites and then into oat bran mixture, coating evenly and completely. Heat oil in a large skillet, add fillets, and fry until golden, about 3 minutes to a side. Serve with lemon wedges and parsley.

Serves 4

Per serving: 366 cal, 15 g fat, 3 g fiber

Confetti Vegetable Enchiladas

Vegetable cooking spray
2 teaspoons vegetable oil
1 cup chopped onion
1 cup chopped green pepper
3 cloves garlic, peeled and
  minced or pressed
One 16-ounce can black
  beans, rinsed and drained

2 cups fresh corn kernels
  (from about 4 ears)
1 teaspoon cumin
One 12-ounce jar
  medium-strength salsa
8 large flour tortillas
1 cup shredded reduced-fat
  Cheddar cheese

Preheat oven to 350°F.

Coat a 7-by-10-inch baking dish with vegetable cooking spray.

In a large skillet, heat the oil and sauté the onion, green pepper, and garlic until tender. Add beans, corn, cumin, and half the salsa; cook a few minutes. Remove from the heat and mash some of the beans with the back of a spoon.

Fill tortillas with bean mixture, roll up, and place seam side down in prepared baking dish. Spread remaining salsa over filled tortillas, cover, and bake for 15 to 20 minutes. Uncover, top with cheese, and return dish to oven until cheese melts. Serve immediately.

Serves 8

Per serving: 329 cal, 10 g fat, 5 g fiber

Fast preparation tip: Substitute one 17-ounce can whole-kernel corn, rinsed and drained, for fresh corn.

Tricolor Pasta Primavera
With Chicken

One 16-ounce package
  tricolor pasta
2 cups sliced carrots
1 cup chopped onion
2 cups fresh broccoli spears
1 cup sliced red or green
  pepper
1 cup fresh mushrooms,
  sliced
1 cup frozen peas, thawed
1 medium fresh tomato,
  cubed

1½ cups cooked and cubed
  chicken breast

Dressing:
½ cup olive oil
½ cup red wine vinegar
2 teaspoons dried basil
1 teaspoon dried oregano
1 clove garlic, minced
Freshly grated black pepper
  and salt to taste

Cook the pasta in boiling water until just tender. Drain the pasta and rinse under cold water.

Meanwhile, in a nonstick skillet sauté the carrot, onion, broccoli, and pepper in 1 teaspoon olive oil until tender-crisp, stirring frequently. This will take just a few minutes. Remove from heat.

In a small jar mix the ingredients for the dressing. Cover and shake until well blended. In a large serving bowl, combine the cooled pasta, cooked vegetables, mushrooms, peas, tomatoes, and chicken with the dressing. Cover and refrigerate. Serve chilled.

Serves 8

Per serving: 400 cal, 16 g fat, 4 g fiber

Marinated Tomato and Shrimp Pasta

4 medium tomatoes, cubed
¼ cup olive oil
¼ cup red wine vinegar
1 tablespoon chopped fresh
    basil, or ½ teaspoon dried
    basil
1 clove garlic, minced
½ teaspoon freshly ground
    black, or red pepper to
    taste

salt to taste
8 ounces cooked, shelled,
    and deveined medium
    shrimp
1 pound linguine
½ cup freshly grated
    Parmesan cheese

In a bowl, combine the tomatoes, oil, vinegar, basil, garlic, pepper, and salt and toss gently. Stir in the shrimp and tomatoes. Cover and refrigerate 2 hours to marinate.

Cook the linguine to just tender in boiling water. Drain the pasta well, then toss with the cold tomato/shrimp marinade. Sprinkle with Parmesan cheese. May be served warm as described or subsequently chilled and served cold.

Serves 8

Per serving: 332 cal, 10 g fat, 1 g fiber

Quick Chili-Stuffed Potatoes

1 cup Quick Chili (page 150)
2 medium baking potatoes,
scrubbed

1 ounce reduced-fat Cheddar
cheese (optional)

Preheat oven to 450°F.

Bake potatoes for 40 minutes, or until soft. Split each potato lengthwise, score potato flesh with a knife, and spoon ½ cup warmed chili over each potato. Sprinkle with cheese if desired. Return to the oven for 5 minutes, or until cheese melts.

Serves 2

Per serving (without cheese): 349 cal, 6 g fat, 6 g fiber

Greek Beans

1 cup Great Northern beans,
picked over and washed
1 bouquet garni
2 cloves garlic, peeled and
halved
1 medium carrot, peeled and
shredded
1 medium onion, peeled and
chopped

1 stalk celery, chopped
1 tablespoon olive oil
2 cups chicken stock
2 teaspoons chopped fresh
oregano, or 1 teaspoon
dried oregano
1 teaspoon nutmeg
Salt
Freshly ground black pepper

Put the beans in a large saucepan with a large amount of cold water; gently heat to a boil and cook beans for 5 minutes. Cover pot, turn off burner, and let beans stand for 1 hour.* Drain in a

*For more on cooking with dry beans, see page 145.

colander and rinse well. Return the beans to the saucepan, along with the bouquet garni and garlic. Add boiling water to cover, reduce heat, and simmer very gently until beans are nearly tender, about 1 hour. Drain. Remove bouquet garni and garlic.

In a large pot, sauté the carrot, onion, and celery in the olive oil until tender. Add the beans, chicken stock, oregano, and nutmeg, bring to a simmer, and cook 10 minutes. Stir in the salt and liberal amounts of black pepper. Serve hot.

Serves 4

Per serving: 181 cal, 5 g fat, 6 g fiber

Butter Bean Casserole

2 cups shelled fresh butter
  beans or lima beans
1 large onion, peeled and
  finely chopped
2 cloves garlic, peeled and
  minced or pressed
1 teaspoon vegetable oil

1½ cups spaghetti sauce,
  preferably homemade
½ teaspoon cumin
¼ teaspoon turmeric
1 tablespoon chopped fresh
  basil leaves, or 1 teaspoon
  dried basil

Preheat oven to 350°F.

In a saucepan, cover beans with boiling water and simmer for 10 minutes. Drain. Sauté onion and garlic in oil in a skillet until tender. In a casserole, combine the contents of the skillet with the drained beans, the spaghetti sauce, cumin, turmeric, and basil. Mix well and bake 30 minutes.

Serves 4

Per serving: 164 cal, 3 g fat, 8 g fiber

Fast preparation tip: Substitute one 15-ounce can butter beans, drained, for fresh.

Dilled Green Beans

4 cups cut fresh green beans
1 teaspoon mustard seed
1 teaspoon dill seed
1 teaspoon crushed red
  pepper flakes

1 teaspoon dried dill weed
3 cloves garlic, peeled and
  pressed or minced
1 cup white vinegar
⅓ cup sugar

Steam green beans until tender. Spray with cold water, then drain thoroughly. Transfer beans to a bowl and mix in the dill seed, red pepper flakes, dill weed, and garlic.

In a small saucepan, combine vinegar and sugar. Bring to a boil and simmer just until sugar dissolves. Remove from heat, add to beans; cool, cover, and refrigerate. Serve chilled and drained. (This dish may be stored for a few days, but the beans get spicier on standing.)

Serves 4

Per serving: 26 cal, 0 fat, 3 g fiber

Savory Brussels Sprouts

1 pound brussels sprouts
2 tablespoons freshly grated
  Parmesan cheese

¼ teaspoon grated fresh
  orange rind
¼ to ½ teaspoon nutmeg

Remove any yellowed outer leaves from brussels sprouts and cut a cross in the root end of each sprout. Steam sprouts for about 10 minutes, until tender-crisp. Sprinkle cheese, orange rind, and nutmeg over hot sprouts and toss.

Serves 5

Per serving: 39 cal, 1 g fat, 4 g fiber

Pineapple Parsnips

**4 medium parsnips (about 1
pound), scraped**
½ cup crushed pineapple
3 tablespoons pineapple juice

**¼ teaspoon grated orange
peel**
2 teaspoons brown sugar
1 teaspoon margarine

Preheat oven to 350°F.

Quarter parsnips lengthwise and cook in a small amount of
boiling water for about 20 minutes, or until tender.

Combine pineapple, pineapple juice, orange peel, and brown
sugar in a bowl. Transfer drained parsnips to a baking dish, pour
the pineapple mixture over them, and dot with margarine. Cover
and bake for about 30 minutes, basting occasionally.

Serves 4

Per serving: 102 cal, 1 g fat, 4 g fiber

Stir-fried Spinach with
Sesame Seeds

1 tablespoon sesame seeds
1 teaspoon vegetable oil
**1 large onion, peeled and
thinly sliced**
**1 clove garlic, peeled and
minced or pressed**
**1 teaspoon minced fresh
gingerroot**

**1 pound fresh spinach,
washed, drained
thoroughly, and chopped**
2 teaspoons soy sauce
1 teaspoon dry sherry
1 teaspoon water

In a skillet, sauté the sesame seeds in oil until golden (watch them
closely; don't let them get too brown). Carefully remove sesame
seeds and set aside, leaving as much oil as possible in the skillet.

Place onion, garlic, and gingerroot in the skillet, adding a bit more oil if necessary, and stir-fry for 2 minutes. Add chopped spinach and stir-fry about 4 minutes. Combine the soy sauce, sherry, and water, add to the skillet, and stir and toss about 2 minutes longer. Sprinkle with the sesame seeds and serve at once.

Serves 2

Per serving: 93 cal, 1 g fat, 4 g fiber

Orange Sweet Potatoes

1 pound (about 3) sweet potatoes (to make 2 cups mashed)
2 teaspoons margarine

1 tablespoon brown sugar
½ cup orange juice
1 teaspoon grated orange rind

Preheat oven to 425°F.

Bake sweet potatoes for 40 minutes to 1 hour, or until tender. Midway through the baking time, pierce each potato deeply with a fork to prevent their bursting. Peel baked potatoes and mash with the margarine. Dissolve the brown sugar in the orange juice and add the orange rind. Mix juice with the mashed potatoes. Spread in a baking dish and bake 10 to 15 minutes longer. Serve hot.

Serves 6

Per serving: 141 cal, 2 g fat, 3 g fiber

Curried Peas and Carrots

1 cup shelled fresh peas	¼ teaspoon turmeric
1 cup diced carrot	½ teaspoon curry powder
1½ teaspoons olive oil	¼ to ½ teaspoon ground red
½ teaspoon minced fresh	pepper
gingerroot	

Blanch peas and carrots separately in boiling water until they are nearly tender. Drain. In a skillet, heat olive oil and sauté gingerroot briefly. Add peas, carrots, turmeric, curry powder, and red pepper, and sauté the mixture 5 to 7 minutes, until vegetables are crisp-tender. Serve hot, by itself or over brown rice, bulgur, or couscous.

Serves 4

Per serving: 53 cal, 2 g fat, 3 g fiber

Fast preparation tip: Substitute one 10-ounce package frozen peas and carrots for fresh.

Lemon Vegetables

2 cups thinly sliced carrots	1 teaspoon snipped fresh dill,
1 clove garlic, peeled and	or ½ teaspoon dried dill
minced or pressed	weed
1 tablespoon olive oil	½ teaspoon freshly grated
2 cups thinly sliced zucchini	lemon rind
1 tablespoon freshly	
squeezed lemon juice	

In a nonstick skillet, sauté carrots and garlic in oil for a few minutes, until carrots brighten in color. Add zucchini and sauté until vegetables are tender-crisp. Stir lemon juice into vegetables, toss them with dill, and add lemon rind.

Serves 6

Per serving: 49 cal, 2 g fat, 2 g fiber

Winter Vegetable Sauté

2 cups carrots, peeled and
  sliced
1 cup broccoli florets
1 cup cauliflower florets
1 cup onion, peeled and
  sliced

1 tablespoon olive oil
1 to 2 teaspoons dried
  rosemary
½ teaspoon paprika

Blanch the carrots, broccoli, and cauliflower separately in boiling water to cover (they should still be quite crisp). Drain well. In a large skillet, sauté the onion in olive oil until it begins to soften. Add the rosemary and blanched vegetables and sauté until tender-crisp. Sprinkle with paprika and serve.

Serves 8

Per serving: 43 cal, 2 g fat, 2 g fiber

Four-Bean Salad

2 cups cut fresh green beans
One 16-ounce can red kidney
beans, drained
One 16-ounce can white
kidney beans or cannellini
beans, drained
One 15-ounce can garbanzo
beans, drained
1 red onion, peeled, thinly
sliced, and separated into
rings

Sweet and Sour Dressing
⅓ cup olive oil
¼ cup white vinegar
¼ cup freshly squeezed
lemon juice
1 tablespoon sugar
Freshly ground black pepper

Quickly blanch fresh green beans in boiling water to cover until tender-crisp. Drain, spray with plenty of cold water, and drain again. Combine drained beans, red, white, and garbanzo beans, and onion rings in large salad bowl.

Mix all dressing ingredients in a blender. Taste for sweetness. Toss salad ingredients with the sweet and sour dressing and refrigerate for several hours or overnight to blend flavors.

Serves 16

Per serving (with dressing): 128 cal, 5 g fat, 3 g fiber

Fast preparation tip: Substitute one 16-ounce can green beans (not French cut), drained, for fresh beans.

Kidney Bean Salad

One 16-ounce can kidney
  beans, drained and rinsed
1 clove garlic, peeled and
  minced or pressed
1 bay leaf

1 tablespoon chopped fresh
  savory leaves, or 2
  teaspoons dried savory
Freshly ground black pepper
1 tablespoon Italian dressing

Mix beans with garlic, bay leaf, and savory. Generously grind black pepper over the mixture and toss everything with the dressing. Chill for several hours to blend flavors. Remove bay leaf before serving.

Serves 4

Per serving: 130 cal, 2 g fat, 3 g fiber

Garbanzo Bean Salad

One 15-ounce can garbanzo
  beans, rinsed and drained
½ cup chopped green pepper
½ cup chopped red pepper
½ cup chopped onion
1½ tablespoons olive oil
1½ tablespoons red wine
  vinegar
1 teaspoon chopped fresh
  oregano leaves, or ½
  teaspoon dried oregano

1 tablespoon chopped fresh
  basil leaves, or ½ teaspoon
  dried basil
½ teaspoon chopped fresh
  thyme, or ¼ teaspoon
  dried thyme
1 teaspoon sugar
Salt and freshly ground
  black pepper to taste

Mix garbanzo beans, green and red peppers, and onion in a salad bowl. Combine oil, vinegar, herbs, sugar, salt, and pepper and pour over vegetables. Toss to blend. Marinate for several hours in the refrigerator before serving.

Serves 6

Per serving: 130 cal, 5 g fat, 2 g fiber

Broccoli, Orange, and Red Pepper Salad

1 cup broccoli spears
2 tablespoons fresh orange
  juice
½ teaspoon sesame oil
1 large orange, peeled and
  sectioned

1 large red bell pepper,
  cored, seeded, and
  julienned

Place broccoli in shallow microwave dish, cover, and cook until tender-crisp, about 5 to 8 minutes on 100 percent.* Mix orange juice and oil. Combine all ingredients with broccoli and microwave again for 1 to 2 minutes. Serve hot.

Serves 4

Per serving: 44 cal, 1 g fat, 3 g fiber

Alternative: Steam broccoli spears for 5 minutes. Add red pepper and orange sections and continue steaming for 3 to 5 minutes.

Meanwhile, mix together the orange juice and sesame oil. When vegetables are tender-crisp, transfer to a serving dish and drizzle with the orange juice mixture. Serve hot.

Spinach Salad

1 cup spinach leaves, washed
and torn
½ cup lettuce leaves, washed
and torn

1 tomato, cut into wedges
½ cup mushrooms, sliced
1 sliced hard-boiled egg

Toss lettuce and spinach together. Arrange tomato wedges, mushrooms, and egg on top. Serve with your favorite dressing.

Serves 1

Per serving (without dressing): 129 cal, 6 g fat, 3 g fiber

Oriental Salad

2 carrots, peeled and thinly
sliced
½ small cucumber, peeled
and julienned
1 large white turnip, peeled
and julienned
4 scallions, both tops and
bulbs, sliced

½ cup white vinegar
1½ tablespoons brown sugar
½ teaspoon fresh gingerroot,
minced
1 teaspoon salt

Put vegetables in a glass or pottery bowl. Bring vinegar, sugar, gingerroot, and salt to a boil in a small saucepan. Pour hot liquid over vegetables and toss. Let stand until mixture reaches room temperature, then chill.

Serves 4

Per serving: 42 cal, 1 g fat, 2 g fiber

Fast Spanish Rice

One 14½-ounce can stewed
  tomatoes, with juice
1½ cups chicken broth
1¼ cups raw brown rice
1 green pepper, cored,
  seeded, and diced

2 teaspoons chili powder
2 teaspoons chopped fresh
  oregano, or 1 teaspoon
  dried oregano
1 clove garlic, peeled and
  minced or pressed

In a saucepan, bring all ingredients to a boil. Reduce heat, cover, and simmer 45 to 50 minutes, or until rice is tender.

Serves 6

Per serving: 125 cal, 1 g fat, 2 g fiber

Brown Rice Pilaf

1 teaspoon vegetable oil
1 small onion, peeled and
  finely chopped
1 rib celery, diced
1 cup fresh mushrooms,
  sliced

1 teaspoon freshly grated
  lemon rind
2 cups chicken or beef stock
1 cup raw brown rice
Chopped fresh parsley

Heat oil in nonstick saucepan and sauté onion, celery, and mushrooms over medium heat until onions are golden. Add lemon rind and stock and bring to a boil. Stir in rice. Cover, reduce heat to very low, and simmer until liquid is absorbed and rice is tender, about 45 to 50 minutes. Remove from heat, fluff pilaf with a fork, and garnish with chopped parsley.

Serves 4

Per serving: 138 cal, 2 g fat, 2 g fiber

Wild Rice and Barley Pilaf

½ cup wild rice
2 cups chicken stock
1 medium carrot, peeled and
  shredded
⅓ cup pearl barley
½ cup sliced fresh
  mushrooms

⅓ cup minced onion
½ teaspoon crushed fresh
  sage, or ¼ teaspoon dried
  crushed sage
Freshly ground black pepper
  to taste
Chopped fresh parsley

Rinse wild rice and drain well. In saucepan, bring to a boil all ingredients except parsley. Reduce heat, cover, and simmer 50 minutes to 1 hour, until rice and barley are tender and liquid is absorbed. Fluff the pilaf with a fork and garnish with abundant chopped parsley.

Serves 6

Per serving: 108 cal, 1 g fat, 2 g fiber

Herbed Barley

½ medium onion, peeled and
  chopped
2 teaspoons vegetable oil
2 cups chicken stock
1 cup medium pearl barley
1 teaspoon chopped fresh
  thyme, or ½ teaspoon
  dried thyme

Salt and freshly ground
  black pepper to taste
2 teaspoons chopped fresh
  parsley

In a saucepan, sauté onion in oil until tender, stirring often. Add stock, barley, thyme, and salt and pepper. Bring to a boil, decrease heat, cover, and simmer about 30 to 35 minutes, until liquid is absorbed and barley is tender. Sprinkle with chopped parsley and serve at once.

Serves 8

Per serving: 108 cal, 2 g fat, 3 g fiber

Bulgur Pilaf

2 teaspoons minced onion
1 clove garlic, peeled and
  minced
2 teaspoons vegetable oil
½ cup raw bulgur
¾ cup chicken stock

1 teaspoon chopped fresh
  oregano leaves, or ½
  teaspoon dried oregano
Salt and freshly ground
  black pepper to taste

In a nonstick skillet, sauté onion and garlic in oil until golden. Add bulgur and sauté, stirring occasionally, for 1 minute. Add chicken stock, oregano, salt, and pepper. Reduce heat, cover, and simmer 12 to 15 minutes, until liquid is absorbed.

Serves 3

Per serving: 74 cal, 4 g fat, 4 g fiber

Polenta

2 cups water
½ cup yellow cornmeal
Dash garlic powder

½ tablespoon grated
Parmesan cheese

In a heavy saucepan, bring 1½ cups water to a boil. Meanwhile, stir ½ cup cold water into cornmeal and add garlic powder. When water in saucepan boils, stir in cornmeal mixture. Turn heat to low and cook, stirring slowly and continually, until mixture is thick and bubbly. Transfer to shallow bowl and sprinkle with cheese. Serve with baked beans for fiber.

Serves 3 to 4

Per serving (without beans): 77 cal, 1 g fat, 0 g fiber

Apricot-Bran Muffins

1 egg
1 cup buttermilk
¼ cup packed brown sugar
2 tablespoons vegetable oil
1 cup bran cereal
1 cup flour

1¼ teaspoons baking powder
1 teaspoon ground cinnamon
½ teaspoon nutmeg
¼ teaspoon baking soda
½ cup diced dried apricots

Preheat oven to 400°F.

Beat egg in a bowl, then add buttermilk, brown sugar, and oil. Stir in cereal and let stand 5 minutes. In another bowl, combine the remaining ingredients, tossing to coat the apricots. Mix wet ingredients with dry ingredients until the latter are just moistened. Fill greased muffin tins ⅔ full and bake for 15 to 20 minutes.

Batter may be covered and refrigerated in an airtight container for up to 7 days.

Makes 14

Per serving (1 muffin): 102 cal, 3 g fat, 2 g fiber

Oat Bran Zucchini Muffins

½ cup unbleached
   all-purpose flour
½ cup whole wheat flour
1 cup oat bran
1 tablespoon baking powder
½ teaspoon cinnamon
¼ teaspoon freshly grated
   nutmeg

⅓ cup firmly packed brown
   sugar
3 egg whites, lightly beaten
¾ cup skim milk
¼ cup safflower oil
1 cup grated zucchini
½ cup coarsely chopped
   walnuts

Preheat oven to 400°F. Oil bottoms of 12 large muffin cups.

Combine flours, oat bran, baking powder, cinnamon, nutmeg, and brown sugar in a large bowl. Mix egg whites, milk, oil, zucchini, and walnuts in a separate bowl. Add zucchini mixture to flour mixture and stir until dry ingredients are thoroughly moistened but batter is still a little lumpy. Fill muffin cups ⅔ full and bake for 20 to 25 minutes.

Makes 12

Per serving (1 muffin): 164 cal, 8 g fat, 1 g fiber

Bake 'Em As You Need 'Em Bran Muffins

3 cups unprocessed wheat
  bran
1 cup boiling water
½ cup (1 stick) margarine
1 cup brown sugar

2 eggs
2½ cups enriched flour
2½ teaspoons baking soda
1 teaspoon salt
2 cups buttermilk

Preheat oven to 400°F.

Combine 1 cup bran and 1 cup boiling water in a bowl, stir, and let steep. In a large bowl, cream margarine and brown sugar. Beat in eggs thoroughly. Sift flour, baking soda, and salt onto wax paper. Add sifted dry ingredients, the steeped bran, and the remaining 2 cups bran to the creamed ingredients, and mix well. Let batter stand about 12 hours before baking. Store it in the refrigerator in a tightly covered container for 2 to 3 weeks.

Fill greased muffin tins ⅔ full and bake for 20 minutes (a bit longer if the batter is cold).

Makes 48

Per serving (1 muffin): 69 cal, 2 g fat, 2 g fiber

Oatmeal Pancakes

⅓ cup whole wheat flour
⅓ cup unbleached
   all-purpose flour
⅓ cup quick-cooking oatmeal
1 tablespoon sugar
1 teaspoon baking powder

½ teaspoon baking soda
¼ teaspoon salt (optional)
1 egg
1 cup buttermilk
1 tablespoon vegetable oil

Mix dry ingredients in a large bowl. In a medium bowl, lightly beat egg and mix with buttermilk and oil. Add the wet ingredients to the dry ingredients and mix until blended. Heat a nonstick griddle over medium heat. Turn the heat down to moderately low and cook the pancakes until the bottoms are brown and the tops start to bubble. Flip them over and cook until the second sides are also brown. Serve immediately.

Makes 10 to 12 pancakes

Per pancake: 71 cal, 3 g fat, 1 g fiber

Rhubarb Cake

1 cup enriched all-purpose
   flour
1 cup whole wheat flour
1 teaspoon baking powder
½ teaspoon baking soda
½ teaspoon cinnamon
¼ teaspoon ground cloves
½ cup (1 stick) margarine
½ cup packed brown sugar
¼ cup white sugar

1 egg
1 teaspoon vanilla
1 cup buttermilk
2 cups (about ½ pound)
   finely diced rhubarb

Topping
¼ cup brown sugar
2 teaspoons cinnamon
½ cup chopped walnuts

Preheat oven to 350°F. Grease a 9-by-13-inch ovenproof glass or enameled baking pan.

Combine the flours, baking powder, baking soda, cinnamon, and cloves on a large piece of wax paper. In a large bowl, cream margarine with brown and white sugars. Add egg and vanilla, and beat mixture until fluffy. Add flour mixture and buttermilk alternately, beating until smooth and well blended. Stir in the rhubarb and pour into the prepared pan.

Mix topping ingredients and sprinkle evenly over the batter. Bake for about 40 minutes, or until cake begins to pull away from the sides of the pan.

Serves 15

Per serving: 196 cal, 9 g fat, 2 g fiber

Peach Crisp

4 cups sliced fresh peaches
1 teaspoon almond extract
1 cup oat bran
½ cup rolled oats
⅓ cup brown sugar

½ cup whole wheat flour
½ teaspoon cinnamon
½ cup (1 stick) chilled
   margarine

Preheat oven to 375°F. Lightly oil an 8-inch ovenproof glass or enameled baking dish.

Spread peaches in baking dish and sprinkle with almond extract. Combine oat bran, rolled oats, brown sugar, flour, and cinnamon in a bowl. With a pastry blender or two knives, cut in margarine until mixture resembles coarse crumbs. Sprinkle topping mixture evenly over peaches. Bake for 35 minutes, or until topping is lightly browned.

8 servings

Per serving: 194 cal, 8 g fat, 4 g fiber

Winter Fruit Compote

2½ cups water
2 tablespoons sugar
1 teaspoon ground cinnamon
3 whole cloves
2 tablespoons freshly
   squeezed lemon juice
¾ cup dried apricots

¾ cup dried prunes
¾ cup cranberries
1 orange, peeled, sectioned,
   and cubed
½ cup raisins
1 tablespoon Cointreau or
   triple sec

Mix the water, sugar, cinnamon, cloves, and lemon juice in a large saucepan and bring to a boil. Reduce heat and add the dried apricots and prunes; cover and simmer gently for 12 minutes. Add the cranberries, diced orange, and raisins, and simmer another 5 minutes. Turn off heat, stir in the Cointreau or triple sec. Serve hot, with yogurt if desired.

Serves 6

Per serving: 114 cal, 1 g fat, 2 g fiber

Minted Pears

2 cups sugar
2 cups water
6 medium pears, peeled,
   cored, and quartered

¼ teaspoon mint extract
1 tablespoon clear crème de
   menthe
Sprigs of fresh mint

In a heavy saucepan, combine sugar and water; stir and cook over medium heat until sugar dissolves, about 2 minutes. Add pears and simmer, uncovered, stirring occasionally, until pears are tender, about 15 minutes. Remove from heat and stir in the mint extract and crème de menthe. Cool pears in the syrup. Garnish each serving with mint sprigs.

Serves 8

Per serving: 266 cal with 4 tablespoons of syrup, 1 g fat, 3 g fiber

Oatmeal Cookies

¾ cup (1½ sticks) margarine
¾ cup firmly packed brown
  sugar
½ cup granulated sugar
1 egg
1 teaspoon vanilla
¾ cup whole wheat flour

¾ cup all-purpose flour
1 teaspoon baking soda
1 teaspoon cinnamon
½ teaspoon nutmeg
3 cups uncooked
  quick-cooking oatmeal

Preheat oven to 375°F. Grease cookie sheets.

Cream margarine and sugars until fluffy. Beat in egg and vanilla. Combine flours, baking soda, and spices. Add flour mixture to egg mixture and mix well. Stir in oats.

Drop by rounded tablespoonfuls on the greased cookie sheets and bake for 8 to 10 minutes. Cool cookies 1 minute on cookie sheets before removing to racks. Store tightly covered.

Makes 4 dozen

Per cookie: 80 cal, 3 g fat, 1 g fiber

10

Now is the Time to Discover Fiber Power!

It's not easy to change deeply ingrained eating habits that have been a part of our daily lives for decades. We're used to certain foods at certain times of the day; some things we've learned to like, and others we've come to dislike.

For example, many people have developed a deep desire for the smooth taste of fat in regular ice cream or for the juicy taste of a piece of beef or lamb. Others feel they need a regular "oral injection" of chocolate or a high-fat dessert.

Of course, none of these foods are high in fiber. Furthermore, they contain saturated fats, cholesterol, and other ingredients that are associated with various health- and life-threatening conditions, such as heart disease and cancer.

How do you change these food cravings and poor nutritional habits that pose such danger to your future? The answer is twofold.

First, focus on the *positive* process of *substituting* high-fiber foods for those that are not high in fiber. If you dwell on the negative—such as by saying, "I've got to stop eating all those gooey desserts,'' or ''I've got to limit myself to one small helping of that meat''—you'll most likely fail. But if you prepare, serve, and eat first those high-fiber foods that are best for your health, the chances are there just won't be much room for the bad dishes.

Second, commit yourself to a full-fiber diet for a few weeks. Many people will simply never get started on a new eating regimen if they think they have to stay on it indefinitely, or worse, for the rest of their lives. They think, ''I'm eventually going to start eating better, but *today* I'll enjoy myself. I'll begin tomorrow.''

Unfortunately, tomorrow rarely comes. If the person does actually embark on a new food plan, he will typically become disillusioned in the first few days. The reason? The new foods taste too unusual, or somehow they don't satisfy deeply entrenched food cravings.

That's why I suggest that you commit yourself to a full-fiber diet for just a few weeks. You can always tell yourself that you can go back to your old ways once your goal of, say, thirty days has been reached. A limited goal always seems more manageable than an unlimited one.

Even more important, dieters will frequently find that they can establish new habits if they just stick with a program for three to four weeks. By the end of that period, tastes begin to change and other factors begin to provide support for the new way of eating.

For example, I've heard many people who cut back on their fat consumption—and stayed with the change for at least a thirty-day period—say, ''I don't really like fats any more. Food with a lot of fat somehow feels oily or unappetizing in my mouth.''

Others become enthusiastic about a change involving regular, easier bowel movements; or a lowering of their cholesterol (which can change dramatically in just one month on a low-fat diet); or the loss of several pounds of body fat. With these benefits to their health and appearance, they find they don't want to return to their old way of eating. The changes themselves become a positive reinforcement for the change to a full-fiber diet.

In this book, you have all the tools you need to effect a significant *and* appetizing transformation of your way of eating. As you proceed, though, be sure to keep your plan simple and practical.

As I've said before, there are many questions that remain to be answered about fiber, and a great deal is still unknown about how the fiber content of various foods operates in the body. But one thing we do know: Regardless of the physiologic mechanisms, *fiber works!* It works in lowering the risk of many diseases, and if you'll just continue to make high-fiber foods the cornerstone of your daily menus, you'll benefit greatly from this food.

In future years, more will become known about the chemical composition and biological impact of fiber. When that happens, we'll most likely add to our store of knowledge such information as

• The *exact* way that fiber helps prevent colon and perhaps other cancers.

When we have a more comprehensive understanding of how fiber combats colon cancer, we may be in a position to apply that knowledge in the fight against other cancers. Among other things, there is hope in the medical research community that certain types of high-fiber diets may be protective against cancers of the pancreas and stomach.

• How fiber can be *prescribed* to treat various diseases and conditions.

We may discover how specific amounts or extracts of certain components of fiber can be used as preventive measures or treatments. Fiber or fiber extracts may become a prevalent form of medication—a nutritional prescription to treat cardiovascular disease, cancer, diabetes mellitus, and other diseases.

• The ways fiber and its ingredients interact with other types of food.

We already know that certain types of fiber can make the zinc or iron in other foods less available to the body. For example, purified cellulose (found in wheat bran) and pectin (found in apples) don't bind iron—that is, make it ineffective in the body—as much as lignin and hemicellulose do.

The more we understand how different types of fiber interact with various vitamins, minerals, and other nutrients, the better we'll be able to maximize the benefits from the food on our tables.

• A comprehensive listing for the general public of the subcomponents of high-fiber foods—and the precise health benefits of those subcomponents.

We know enough now to recommend the consumption of various kinds of fiber as part of a general preventive medicine plan. As you've seen, we're aware that insoluble fibers are associated with a lower risk of colon cancer. Also, soluble fibers have been linked to lower cholesterol levels.

But there's so much more to learn! When research on fiber progresses further, as it surely will in the next couple of decades, I expect that the basic tools you've learned in this book will still be valid. But they will form only a basic foundation for the application of a much more exact science in your kitchen. Today's fiber prescriptions will become tomorrow's fiber way of life.

Index

191

Myron Winick, M.D., is currently R.R. Williams Professor of Nutrition (Emeritus), Columbia University College of Physicians and Surgeons. From 1972–1990, Dr. Winick was Director of the Institute of Human Nutrition at Columbia University College of Physicians and Surgeons. He is the recipient of the Osborne and Mendel Award for Research in Nutrition from the American Institute of Nutrition (1976), and the Agnes Higgins Award from the March of Dimes for Research in Maternal Nutrition (1983). The author of a number of books, Dr. Winick has been a member of numerous scientific committees and boards including the Food and Nutrition Board of the National Research Council (1983–1989), the Nutrition Committee of the American Academy of Pediatrics, and the Nutrition Study Section of the National Institute of Health. Dr. Winick is married to Elaine Lasky Winick and they have two sons, Jonathan and Stephen.

William Proctor is a graduate of Harvard College and Law School and a former writer and reporter for the New York *Daily News*. He has authored, co-authored, or ghostwritten more than 60 books, including several bestsellers, on such topics as fitness, nutrition, medicine, and religion. He lives with his wife Pam and son Michael in New York City.